Prais

HOPE FOR THE BEST, PLAN FOR THE REST

"This is a much-needed book. The authors offer an engaging, positive, and helpful set of principles to people who are sick, their close supporters, and those who want to help them navigate the challenge of serious illness—including dying—their way. This book is like a conversation with a wise coach on adapting the system so that health care is tailored to your individual preferences. *Hope for the Best, Plan for the Rest* is kind, clear, and system-changing: a clarion call for a patient-led revolution in health care."

KATHRYN MANNIX, MD, palliative care physician and *Sunday Times*–bestselling author of *With the End in Mind* and *Listen*

"A lightning bolt of hope! This book shows patients and families struggling with serious illness how to get the honest, personalized care they need. *Hope for the Best, Plan for the Rest* is a palliative care tour de force and essential reading for all who feel overwhelmed and alone in the health care system, along with the clinicians who care for them."

THERESA BROWN, RN, *New York Times*–bestselling author of *Healing* and *The Shift*

"*Hope for the Best, Plan for the Rest* offers succinct, practical tips for getting the best care and living well through the course of your illness."

IRA BYOCK, MD, palliative care physician and bestselling author of *The Four Things That Matter Most* and *The Best Care Possible*

"Shout it from the rooftops, the Waiting Room Revolution has begun! With Drs. Sammy Winemaker and Hsien Seow leading the charge, no patient or family member will face illness with their eyes wide shut ever again!"

HARVEY MAX CHOCHINOV, MD, author of *Dignity Therapy* and *Dignity in Care*

"Drs. Sammy Winemaker and Hsien Seow are leading a revolution—one we all need to be a part of! Get planning! Their decades of research, as well as clinical and lived experience, are compiled here to provide readers with essential keys to navigating illness. Do yourself a favor: read this book and make sure your family and friends do too!"

KATHY KORTES-MILLER, PhD, author of *Talking about Death Won't Kill You*

"This rigorous and compassionate book—the result of two thought leaders' experiences in research and medical practice—helps to dispel the chaos and uncertainty of receiving a new and life-changing diagnosis. Drs. Sammy Winemaker and Hsien Seow are wise and relentless guides who offer practical and hard-won advice that will empower people to take charge of their health and destiny no matter what they face."

SUNITA PURI, MD, palliative care physician and author of *That Good Night*

"*Hope for the Best, Plan for the Rest* offers a fresh, welcome, and long-overdue opportunity for all of us to think and act differently when challenged by a diagnosis. Its insights and suggestions are valuable for patients, families, and health care professionals alike. The easy, personal style of this book makes it a great companion for anyone who must journey through a difficult time of uncertainty and fear. I recommend it wholeheartedly."

HEATHER RICHARDSON, RN, PhD, director of education, research, and end of life policy at St Christopher's Hospice, London, UK

"An essential read, full of practical tools for those who are newly diagnosed, engaged in caregiving, or simply want to support someone with compassion. *Hope for the Best, Plan for the Rest* shows you how to amplify your voice, access the best possible care, and best prepare for your future health care needs—your way. This book is like having your own personal health care mentor at your side, teaching you how to have honest, open conversations with your needs front and center."

LAUREL L. GILLESPIE, MBA, CHE, CEO of the Canadian Hospice Palliative Care Association

HOPE
FOR THE BEST
PLAN
FOR THE REST

PAGE TWO

HOPE FOR THE BEST PLAN FOR THE REST

7 Keys for Navigating a Life-Changing Diagnosis

DR. SAMMY WINEMAKER
DR. HSIEN SEOW

Some names and identifying details have been changed to protect the privacy of individuals.

This book is not intended as a substitute for the medical advice of physicians. The reader should regularly consult a physician in matters relating to his/her/their health and particularly with respect to any symptoms that may require diagnosis or medical attention.

Figures 1–4 (on pages 59–61) are adapted with permission from J. Lynn and D.M. Adamson, *Living Well at the End of Life: Adapting Health Care to Serious Chronic Illness in Old Age* (RAND Health report WP-137, 2003), doi.org/10.7249/WP137.

Cataloguing in publication information is available from Library and Archives Canada.
ISBN 978-1-77458-296-1 (paperback)
ISBN 978-1-77458-297-8 (ebook)

Page Two
pagetwo.com

Edited by Kendra Ward
Copyedited by Steph VanderMeulen
Proofread by Alison Strobel
Cover, interior design, and illustrations by Jennifer Lum
Printed and bound in Canada by Friesens
Distributed in Canada by Raincoast Books
Distributed in the US and internationally by Macmillan

23 24 25 26 27 6 5 4 3 2

waitingroomrevolution.com

To our mothers and fathers, who gave us wings.

To our spouses, who empowered us to fly.

And to our daughters, who taught us to enjoy the view.

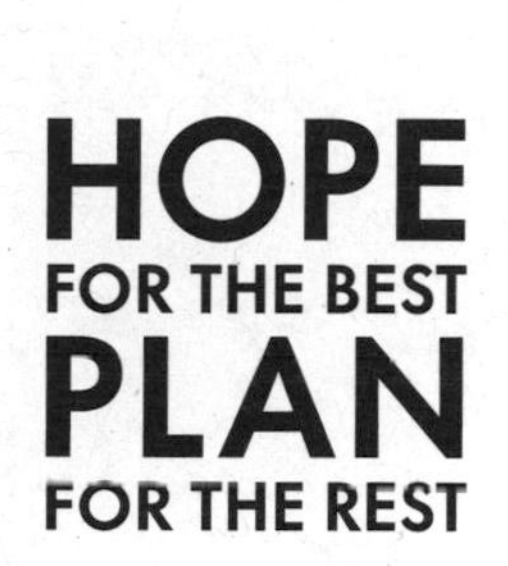
HOPE
FOR THE BEST
PLAN
FOR THE REST

CONTENTS

PREFACE

DEAR READER,

I applaud you for opening this book. You may not realize how important it is that you have taken the step to delve deeper into the major health situation you find yourself in. Seeking out knowledge is the most valuable step you can take to obtain more control and choice moving forward. This book will help you understand why.

You're probably reading this because you, or someone close to you, received a life-changing diagnosis. It is understandable if you feel scared, angry, sad, confused, helpless . . . or all of the above. You may worry that nothing in your life will ever be the same.

I am here to tell you there *is* hope.

Of the thousands of patients with serious illnesses whom I have cared for, I've met two groups: those who are in control, prepared, and "in the know"; and those who are overwhelmed, frustrated, and "in the dark." The illness experiences of these two groups are completely opposite. The former learned about the big picture of their illness, planned ahead, and received care that matched their preferences. Their experience was more proactive and empowering.

The second group got stuck in the day-to-day of their illness, and always seemed to be two steps behind, reactive, and feeling lost. With this latter group of patients, I typically spend hours filling in missing information about the changing nature of their illness so they can make knowledgeable decisions and plan ahead. They often say to me, "I wish I'd known that sooner."

I spent years investigating the difference between the overwhelmed patient and the prepared patient. In the end, I discovered seven keys that every patient should learn about when they are diagnosed. I call them "keys" because they unlock the secrets that help people navigate the role of a patient. These keys are easy to use and can be applied immediately.

1. **Walk Two Roads.** People naturally want to stay positive throughout their illness and not give up. You walk two roads by maintaining hope during the twists and turns of your illness while seeking truthful information to stay grounded.

2. **Zoom Out.** You may feel uncertain about how things might unfold. By learning to zoom out, you get a road map for what to expect in the long view of an illness.

3. **Know Your Style.** Some people feel helpless because the biology of a diagnosis cannot be changed. But by knowing your style—how you have lived your life, your unique way of being, your past experiences—you can harness this information to gain more control of your illness journey.

4. **Customize Your Order.** At times, you may feel less like a person and more like a numbered object on a health care conveyor belt. When you know how to customize your order, you can better maintain your sense of self.

5 **Anticipate Ripple Effects.** Even though you rightfully are at the center of your illness, people around you will be involved in and impacted by your care. You can learn to anticipate ripple effects so those around you can support you fully and be supported themselves.

6 **Connect the Dots.** You will interact with health care providers in a complex, disconnected system with its own culture and language. You can learn how to ensure vital information about you doesn't fall through the cracks.

7 **Invite Yourself.** If you are intimidated by the power imbalance between you and health care providers, you may find it hard at times to speak up. I'll show you how and when to invite yourself into the conversation so you get the vital, but often hidden, information that you deserve to know. After all, information is power, especially when you have it early in your illness journey.

This book is filled with hope. Although I cannot change that you received a life-changing diagnosis, I hope to improve your experience living with it. By using the seven keys, I hope to transform your illness journey from being in the dark to being in the know, where you never have to say, "I wish I had known that sooner."

Sincerely,

Dr. Sammy

INTRODUCTION

NOT TOO long ago, I was asked to make a home visit to meet Gerry, a fifty-eight-year-old man with idiopathic pulmonary fibrosis, a progressive lung disease that carries an average life expectancy of three to six years after diagnosis. Gerry's lung disease remained remarkably stable for the first two years. Then he began to notice a decline. He experienced more shortness of breath and needed higher amounts of oxygen. His stamina diminished each month. A special respirology team had followed him for three years before I met him. When he worsened, the team told Gerry that without a lung transplant, he would die from his illness. He latched on to the possibility of a transplant; he felt great hope for the future. But he kept getting worse. In his last appointment with this respirologist, he heard devastating news: his disease had advanced too far for him to be eligible for a transplant. With that, his hopes were dashed. He felt he had no choice but to request Medical Assistance in Dying, which was legalized in Canada in 2016. In other countries, this request is called physician-assisted death or euthanasia. Without any specialized respirology treatment available, Gerry was transferred back to his family doctor, who hadn't seen him in years and was unaware of his advanced condition. This is when his family doctor asked me, a palliative care physician, to meet with Gerry for the first time.

Walking up Gerry's front porch, I took a deep breath to steady myself. Gerry's wife answered the door. She seemed agitated, as if she'd been pacing in anticipation of my arrival.

"Before you come in, Dr. Winemaker, I need you to know that we don't want anyone blocking his request for Medical Assistance in Dying," she said.

I hadn't even crossed the threshold of the front entrance, but her anxiety was palpable during this brief, intense shakedown of my intention. I assured her I was there to support Gerry and her through this journey and to provide a palliative care consult, not to change anyone's mind. I told her, as I do many of my patients with a life-limiting illness, that my role as a palliative care physician is to help Gerry live as well as he can for as long as he can.

As she led me to the living room of their cozy home, I noticed a few family photos hanging in the hallway and a lace tablecloth on the large wooden dining table. The scent of a vanilla candle wafted from the kitchen. Gerry sat cross-legged on a leather couch facing a bay window. This is typical of people who are breathless. They naturally position themselves in front of a window with a view. An open vista, especially one with leaves moving gently in the breeze, calms the mind with a sense of air and breath. Wearing an oxygen mask on his face, Gerry looked emaciated, his skin sallow. Despite his fast and shallow breathing through the oxygen mask, he smiled and warmly welcomed me.

I sat down and asked him to share his story. I soon realized that over the course of his illness no one had told him what to expect as he grew sicker. Around his initial diagnosis, he was told that his lung disease was not curable and that he would eventually die from it if he didn't get a transplant. That was it. He knew of nothing beyond tests, treatments, and a possible transplant. No one had ever sat with him to review the course his disease would take from beginning to middle to end. He also hadn't asked many questions about the what-ifs. When he began to get weaker, the only option offered to him was the possibility of a transplant. He knew nothing about managing his breathlessness or other symptoms, or of the supports available to him and his family while he waited for a transplant. When the devastating news came that he wouldn't get a transplant, Gerry was left to believe that he would suffocate to death. So he requested Medical Assistance in Dying to avoid suffocation. I couldn't blame him.

But there were plenty of other possibilities. I spent more than two hours that morning talking with Gerry and his family. They were shocked to learn that he would not suffocate to death if appropriate care was offered, and that his decline could be gentle until the end.

I asked him, "If your breathing was more comfortable and you could remain independent for longer, would you consider putting off your decision about assisted dying for now?" I wanted a few days to prove to Gerry that a third option was available to him: comfort. Gerry agreed to try medication for his breathlessness. He said he would give me a week to make him feel better.

After I left the house, I got into my car feeling dispirited. I had seven days to do the work that should have begun with his diagnosis. I wasn't trying to convince him to change his mind about assisted dying—that was his choice. But I wanted to fill in all information gaps in his care. He deserved to know everything. It was unfair and inappropriate for Gerry to think that his only choices were suffocation or assisted death.

Gerry tried the medication I prescribed for two days. It worked slowly for him because he needed to start with a low dose to avoid side effects. If this medication had been started earlier, he would have had more time to increase it safely to the right dose. He quickly lost trust in me and arranged for a medically assisted death.

It felt like Gerry's choice for Medical Assistance in Dying had been set in stone even before I had arrived. He didn't choose it because I failed him. He chose it because he was so breathless for so long and he was done living like this.

When I learned of his decision, I sat in my car and wept. I cried all the way to my next patient. I knew the cycle would repeat when I got there: another version of the same heartbreaking challenge of trying to catch up on problems that should've been discussed weeks, months, or years before.

The Lightbulb Moment

A few weeks after my last visit with Gerry, I met my friend and colleague (and now the coauthor of this book) Dr. Hsien Seow for coffee early one morning.

It was a cool autumn day, with gray skies and drizzling rain. I ordered my usual, a medium coffee, and he was already there with his, waiting for me. That morning we were there to talk about a research project focused on palliative care education for health care providers.

When I first met Hsien, I was immediately impressed. He was a superstar health care researcher at McMaster University in Hamilton, Ontario, where I also worked. He had been leading research in end-of-life care for fifteen years and had dozens of grants and publications on the topic. His work had been used by policymakers throughout Canada. Hsien and I shared a burning desire to improve the patient and family experience, not just rack up academic accolades.

I recalled listening to him speak at a conference about the reason he focused on palliative care in his research: his mother had died of cancer when he was younger. He would never forget that the health care team did not prepare him or his family for the possibility that she would die, even though her particular illness had a very predictable decline. They had been utterly unprepared for her death. She received chemotherapy until she died. They never had a chance to say goodbye or find closure. Like me, Hsien was driven by the many patient and family stories of feeling lost throughout the journey, not knowing what to expect next.

"Before we talk about the project, there's something I want to ask you, Sammy," Hsien said to me as I sat down.

I was silent. I sipped my hot coffee.

"Do you ever wonder if our research is making a difference?" he asked.

He confessed to me that he was at a low point in his career. He felt disillusioned because he'd met too many policymakers and health care executives who were more concerned with keeping the status quo than changing things for the better. He doubted that his research would have any impact in the real world.

I was surprised. From the outside, our two careers seemed rather successful. But on the inside, we both felt empty. Somehow, we were both in a dark hour of our professional careers at the same time.

Now, there were many great education programs for health care providers. I had taught some of them for years. High-quality and standardized education is extremely important. But the needle was not moving fast enough. Despite the training, not enough providers were giving palliative care to their patients. Financial and systemic barriers were a big part of the problem.

Over a second cup of coffee, I asked a question that would change everything.

"Why are we doing this education only for physicians? Shouldn't we be teaching patients and families about how to have a better illness experience? After all, they are the people who need this information."

In that lightbulb moment, both Hsien and I saw a possibility for change: shifting the focus from educating health care providers to activating patients and families to take charge of their illness journey. This shift in focus gave us renewed hope that the illness experience could be better and that large-scale change was possible.

The Waiting Room Revolution

This book represents a part of a larger social movement that we call the Waiting Room Revolution. This name suggests the fundamental change we hope to see.

Patients and families spend hundreds of hours traveling to medical appointments and sitting in waiting rooms. The dread, fear, and tension in these rooms are palpable. Patients and families stare at the floor, filled with anxiety as they await the results of their latest imaging. Patients have a word for this: "scanxiety." They wonder if the news ahead will be good or bad. They feel out of control.

More than that, their life stands still as it is dictated by the latest round of information about their condition. People say they feel stuck in a holding pattern—they don't plan too far ahead because they are waiting to see if or when things will change. They *live* in a metaphorical waiting room, too.

So we need a revolution in every waiting room, one in which activated patients and families come to the health care system more aware of their critical role in the illness experience and more prepared to partner with their medical team.

Our movement began with a podcast, also called *The Waiting Room Revolution*. We spoke to guests who had information and tips on how to improve the illness experience. Season 1 focused on the seven keys. And we are excited that the podcast has gained popularity and served as a living lab of our keys with real patients and families.

This led us to writing this book. And though Hsien and I created the revolution together, we decided to write this book in a single-person perspective, from my vantage point as a doctor.

Ultimately, we realized that to create large-scale and massive, sustainable change, we need not just health care providers who openly give information about all serious illnesses, but also patients and families who know how to get the information they need at all points throughout the illness. We want to create a new kind of patient, one who is equipped with the advice of the many patients before them. One who is wise to the barriers that exist, and readied with solutions, skills, and actions to overcome them. We want to activate *you* to be hopeful and prepared right from the start of a life-changing diagnosis.

1

FROM "IN THE DARK" TO "IN THE KNOW"

“We need to stop just pulling people out of the river. We need to go upstream and find out why they’re falling in.”

ARCHBISHOP DESMOND TUTU

AS A PHYSICIAN who makes daily house calls, I have cared for thousands of patients and families who craved more open information about the health care system and their serious illness, right from the time of diagnosis. Like you, they needed and deserved to know how to be hopeful and prepared.

The Seven Keys to a Better Illness Experience

I am a palliative care doctor, which means I care for people who are facing non-curable illnesses that shorten their life expectancy. I have had the privilege of caring for thousands of patients at the end of their illness, in their homes—where they feel at ease to be themselves. This unique vantage point has been unbelievably illuminating. Through their stories, patients often unintentionally shine light on the many earlier failings of our health care system. I have seen how these shortcomings have contributed to unnecessary suffering.

Our health care system is imperfect—some might even say broken. Much of what I do in my daily clinical work is clean up this disarray for patients and families, often almost too late. By the time I meet people in their homes, they are usually at the very end of life, unsure of what to expect, scared of what is coming, and craving honest, open conversations.

Even though lots of information has been communicated to them by many different health care teams, no one has given them a road map of how their illness will unfold. I see firsthand the massive disconnect between what patients and families hear and what doctors and the health care system say. I do my best to decode the system for patients and families, acting like a medical interpreter to make sense of it all.

Although doctors, nurses, and allied health professionals know more about illness and mortality than most people, many are uncomfortable talking openly about the possibility of decline. This begins a pattern of interactions based on half-truths, implied consequences, unspoken questions, and ill-addressed fears. Consequently, patients and their families make many important decisions about treatments, work, and family life with only partial information. This inevitably leads to regret and disappointment.

These realizations of the unintentional harm we cause propelled me to advocate for both health care system change and improvements in the education of health care providers. Eventually, I realized that it wasn't only health care providers who needed more education. Patients and families also craved more open information about how to navigate the system and what to expect in their serious illness. They needed and deserved this information.

This book represents the journey Hsien and I have taken to reverse-engineer the stories of the thousands of patients we have heard, either at the bedside or through our research, and to decipher the differences between "in the know" and "in the dark" experiences. We realized that patients and families often had false assumptions about the health system and their illness. We spent time clearly naming those assumptions and then revealing the hidden realities—the things people didn't know they didn't know. Ultimately, we arrived at seven essential keys that every patient and their family should know at the beginning of a life-changing diagnosis, and that you will learn about in this book:

1. **Walk Two Roads.** Hope for the best, and plan for the rest.
2. **Zoom Out.** Understand the big picture of your illness.
3. **Know Your Style.** Review your past patterns for insights into how you will journey throughout your illness.
4. **Customize Your Order.** Tailor the care plan to your values and preferences.
5. **Anticipate Ripple Effects.** Prepare for how those caring for you will also need to be supported.
6. **Connect the Dots.** Play a central role in coordinating information in the larger system.
7. **Invite Yourself.** Initiate conversations about what to expect and advocate for yourself.

While researching this book, I realized that the keys to a better illness experience are essential skills for every patient, with any kind of condition, not just those who are dying. This is a book about how to live well, be fully informed, and be an activated patient. It can empower you to take back power, control, and choice in your illness experience. It will show you how to feel like a person, not a patient, living with a life-changing illness.

Becoming a Hopeful and Prepared Patient

You didn't choose to become a patient. That label was given to you when you received your diagnosis. You may feel as if there is so much uncertainty and there are so many unknowns about the future. But it is possible to train to be a hopeful and prepared patient.

One of the most important things I can share with you is that you should seek to know the nature of your illness. It is important to establish if you do have a *life-changing* illness. Often, people take their diagnosis at face value and don't realize that there are different types of illnesses that will have a greater or lesser impact on you and your family. Is this an illness that will be cured or not cured? If not cured, will it be life-changing? A life-changing illness meets at least one of these criteria:

- Chronic (in other words, it cannot be fully cured)
- Progressive (it will worsen over time)
- Life-limiting (it will shorten one's life)

Chronic. Some illnesses are chronic, which means they cannot be cured and won't ever fully go away. This includes HIV/AIDS, Crohn's disease, and diabetes. It also includes some mental health disorders and physical disabilities. Because of advances in health care and medications, many of these illnesses can remain stable and controlled for long periods of time. This book will help patients who must navigate their illness and the health system, in some way or another, for the rest of their lives.

Progressive. Some illnesses are progressive, which means they will worsen over time and lead to a decline in health and physical function. This includes illnesses such as osteoarthritis, macular degeneration, and spinal stenosis. Usually, medical treatment and therapy stabilizes the illness for some duration, but eventually the illness worsens and then the quality of life worsens, too. This book will help patients gain more control by empowering them to obtain vital information about what to look for and prepare for to maintain quality of life.

Life-limiting. Some illnesses will also shorten a person's life, which means people eventually die from these diagnoses. Many illnesses fit into this group. They include some types of heart disease, respiratory disease, non-curable cancers, types of liver or kidney failure, neurodegenerative diseases, and frailty. Sometimes there are many, many years in between diagnosis and death. This book can help patients be more hopeful and grounded by activating them to understand the big picture of their illness and make choices about their care that are specific to their goals and values.

The most important part of understanding your illness is an awareness of whether your illness meets any of these three criteria. Knowing if you meet some or all of the criteria sets the tone of your illness journey. What you hope for and what you need to prepare for depend on the nature of your illness.

For example, you don't want to assume your illness is only chronic if it is expected to worsen over time and will shorten your life. Some chronic illnesses can, in fact, shift to become progressive and life-limiting at some stage. For example, diabetes is often thought of as a chronic illness, but over a lifetime it can cause organ damage to the heart and kidneys, which can then shorten one's life. That is why it is important to talk with your doctors about the features of your illness.

However, my experience has been that most people don't exactly know if their diagnosis meets one, two, or all three criteria. They are scared because they know it is a serious diagnosis and place their complete trust in their doctors to help them.

So if you don't know whether your illness will end up being life-changing, I strongly encourage you to ask your health care professionals.

Conversation Starters: Here are some suggestions for questions to ask.

- "Is my illness curable or is it chronic and non-curable? How long should I expect to have this condition?"
- "Will it worsen over time? Even if there are effective treatments, at some point should I expect it to worsen?"
- "Is it possible that the illness will shorten my natural life expectancy? Is this illness life-limiting or life-threatening?"

Uncertain Whether You Want to Know More?

It is understandable if you are hesitant to read on and learn more about your illness. A life-changing diagnosis will cause you to experience a wide variety of emotions at different points throughout your illness. This will look and feel different to everyone. Your emotions will have a dynamic and ongoing interplay with your physical well-being and your ability, at times, to take charge of your illness journey. I appreciate that people need time to adjust, have different levels of readiness for information, and have varying preferences for how much to know.

When you are ready, the information in this book offers one of the most powerful strategies to help you be in the know so you can have a better experience. There are many decisions to make throughout an illness that will affect you, your life, and those you love. The choices you make will depend heavily on the nature of the illness. Therefore, the basic information you should understand is whether your illness meets any of the three criteria—that is, is it chronic, progressive, or life-limiting—and if it will thus be life-changing. Beyond that, how much you want to know is up to you.

However, you should be aware that patients who do not like to look ahead, who would rather not know more and thus avoid asking the big questions, or who are in denial after being told end up having more fear and anxiety about the future, which amplifies other symptoms and causes a great deal of unnecessary suffering for themselves and their loved ones. So if you still aren't sure you want to know, I encourage you to read the rest of this book anyway to learn how to be an informed and empowered patient.

Sometimes people dread the answers to big questions because they are scared or are uncomfortable with uncertainty. But psychology research shows that any information, even tough-to-hear information, is grounding. Even if the news is not what you had hoped for, you *are* resilient. You might need time to adjust to the big news or new information, but you will likely adjust. In the end, I have seen repeatedly that information is the most important medicine.

Tip: Some people assume that if they are receiving treatment, then their condition is curable. Most conditions have a range of treatment options. The treatment's intent may be to cure you, extend your life, maintain your quality of life, or relieve your symptoms. Each of these intents is fundamentally different. Many people do not fully appreciate the purpose of their treatment. If treatments are keeping their symptoms at bay, they may start to believe, mistakenly, that they can be cured of their condition or that the stable state they are feeling will be maintained forever. Don't fall prey to these false assumptions. Understand your illness and the intent of your treatments.

Activating Family and Other Caregivers

This book is for patients, and it is also for patients' families. Most patients have people who are deeply involved in their care. It is rare that a person goes through an illness alone. Throughout this book, I use the term "family" to describe your chosen family, which may or may not be blood-related. Family can be thought of as your inner crew or inner circle, your spouse or life partner, your children or parents. It can include close friends and neighbors.

Like patients, families are along for the illness journey. Before the diagnosis, they were "just" a spouse or partner, a sibling, child, or friend. And suddenly they were given the label of caregiver or carer. They often don't identify with or relate to this new label. They almost always don't fully understand what this role entails. Sometimes they are a caregiver to multiple people.

Caregivers and family members may suffer, too. Many times, a family member of my patients will look back on their experience and tell me they felt stripped of their sense of control, independence, autonomy, and personhood. They felt regretful and angry because they would have made different choices along the way if they'd only known how things were going to play out. They felt robbed of time they would have spent differently. A negative illness experience can leave family members scarred with guilt, resentment, and bitterness for years.

Families need the same information as the patient. Sometimes they might need even more. In the pages to come, you will see some "family shout-outs," where messages are directed at and particularly important for family.

How This Book Is Organized

In the chapters ahead, I outline the seven keys to become a hopeful and prepared patient. In each chapter, I share

- one of the seven keys and three practical actions you can use right away;
- the false assumption that can leave you feeling in the dark and the corresponding reality that can shape a journey in which you are in the know;
- tips, exercises, and conversation starters to apply the keys; and
- with permission, real-life stories of patients I have cared for or interviewed to illustrate the keys (some names have been changed to protect anonymity, where requested).

Note: since all my patients have chronic and progressive and life-limiting illnesses, the patient stories tend to have that flavor. Even if you don't have a life-limiting illness, the stories still offer valuable lessons.

I follow the seven keys with a chapter that includes tips for putting it all together and special consideration for unique populations and circumstances. I also include two chapters specifically for those who have a progressive and life-limiting illness and want a glimpse into the advanced stages of the illness. I present some of the answers to the most common questions asked by patients and families in this late stage of an illness. You may want to read these chapters later, when you feel ready, or avoid them altogether.

This book is about learning to journey through your illness in the know, with your eyes wide open. For many, being a patient is a brand-new role, and it is easy to set off on the wrong foot. Over and over, patients feel in the dark, fall through the cracks, or don't know what they don't know. They end up bobbing around like a boat without an anchor through their illness, which leads to them being totally overwhelmed if there is a storm.

But it doesn't have to be that way. Certain skills will help you extract information and the meaning of that information from the health care system. This will allow you to remain in control, have more choices, provide informed consent, feel empowered, and retain your sense of self. My hope is that you can apply the following seven keys right away so that you're more hopeful and prepared at every stage of your illness.

2

WALK TWO ROADS

“Hope should be the consequence of medicine, not the goal.”

DAVID HENDERSON

THE KEY Walk Two Roads means you hope for the best and plan for the rest. This key teaches you to toggle between staying positive and maintaining faith in medical treatments and seeking honest, accurate information. You keep your eye on the best outcome while considering what to do if things go sideways.

Assumption: You Stay Positive or You Give Up

Most people facing a life-changing diagnosis assume that they have to stay 100 percent positive or else they're giving up hope. People often think that planning ahead means they are giving in to the disease and that by speaking about possible negative outcomes, they are somehow increasing the odds it will happen. Therefore, most patients and families walk a single, narrow road, focusing on being hopeful while ignoring the rest.

It's very common to see my patients surrounded by enthusiastic cheerleaders. My patients usually go along with it because it feels good, particularly at the beginning. Patients and families share with me the blogs and books they've read about the healing powers of positive thinking, ones that urge everyone to believe positive thinking is the best medicine. This is pressure as much as enthusiasm. I have seen patients feel tremendous obligation to stay positive or risk betraying the people supporting them. Health care providers join the cheerleading squad, too. You'll hear doctors or nurses say such things as, "Miracles happen every day" or "There is always something in the cupboard."

Walking the road of hope usually means readying yourself to fight a battle against the disease. You might think, "I have to be strong. I have to battle the disease." I've heard patients say, "I don't want to know any statistics about how bad this is. I just want to know how to beat this." The cheerleading squad of family, friends, and health care providers reinforce the battle cry, telling the patient that they're a fighter who will defy the odds.

Media headlines talk about celebrities "losing the battle to the disease." The implicit messages are that if you die from a disease, you didn't fight hard enough, and that you had a choice in succumbing to the illness. The implication is that the patient alone has the power to win or lose the battle. But this is wrong. It sets up unrealistic hopes and adds to the burden, which can be crushing.

My patients sometimes confide in me that they feel like they must always put on a brave face and think positive thoughts. They feel pressure on all sides—from family, friends, medical and hospital staff, even from the media—to stay positive. Not to give up. From day one, the message is clear: you must be unrelentingly hopeful.

Reality: Hope Is Grounded in Realistic Information

Hope shouldn't mean that you don't plan for the future. Too often, walking the road of unrelenting positivity leads patients and families to be overly optimistic about treatment options. They are not fully aware of whether the illness is curable or chronic, progressive, and/or life-limiting—and they are scared to ask. They don't probe about the reality of their life-changing illness. They shy away from difficult conversations about what happens if things don't go well. Even health care teams, who know what happens over time, often find it easier to say, "Let's hope for the best."

When patients present positive attitudes during visits to the clinic, doctors usually follow their lead. Important information is left unsaid. I've met patients discharged from the heart failure clinic program who think they are doing well when, in fact, they were sent home because treatments could no longer help. I've met patients with end-stage lung disease who are repeatedly admitted to the hospital, stabilized, and sent home, but no one tells them they will never completely bounce back to their old selves, that they will progressively worsen.

I don't want to downplay the scientific medical advances that are being explored to eradicate disease or meaningfully increase quality of life. But these breakthroughs are rarer than they are common. Sometimes a family will try to hide a true diagnosis from a patient for worry that the patient will become depressed. This unspoken charade can go on for inordinate amounts of time.

One of the main reasons more providers and patients don't talk about preparing for the rest is that they worry that talking about different what-if scenarios, including the possibility of death, will rob people of hope and make them depressed and sad. However, research shows that open and honest conversations about the future reduce anxiety and depression. In fact, open, honest discussions may even help people live longer. Certainly, the initial conversations can bring about a range of emotions, but people typically adjust with time and become more grounded with real information.

Staying hopeful and cheerleading have their place. But without a balanced approach, excessive hopefulness can morph into toxic positivity—the excessive overgeneralization of a happy, optimistic state, where people feel obligated to present a positive front. Psychologists recognize that toxic positivity is not a healthy way to deal with challenges. It leads to denial and minimization of reality while invalidating legitimate feelings such as grief or sadness. Often false cheerleading leads to false hope.

Anya's Story: In the Dark

I met Anya, a retired psychotherapist and patient-family advocate, at a caregiver conference. For forty-three years, she was married to Fred, a retired high school teacher and volunteer firefighter. A few years into his retirement, Fred was diagnosed with colon cancer that had spread to his liver. Anya told me they were in the dark throughout the illness. During treatment, she felt they were cogs in a relentless machine. "We could not stop. We didn't even know stopping was an option," she said.

From the start, Anya felt pressure to battle the cancer and only walk the road of hope. She described it as the "tyranny of hope." She felt that everywhere she turned in the cancer center, they had "pumped up the volume on hope." Despite repeated questions, health care providers were unwilling to talk to her or Fred about what happens when treatment fails. Anya told me, "You felt like a bad caregiver or a bad patient if you weren't fighting. You had to fight. Even when you had no energy to fight anymore." The message she was getting loud and clear: "If you die, it's because you didn't fight hard enough. It's your fault."

The only time anyone acknowledged that there was no cure for Fred was at his first appointment, when the oncologist told him to get his affairs in order. From then on, the constant and cheerful refrain was, "There's always something in the cupboard"—a treatment, drug, or clinical trial to buy more time. The health care team was caring but gave false hope. It seemed as though the health care providers were "in complete denial about dying." This cheery optimism left Anya feeling extremely isolated. She did not have the valuable information she wanted, such as how the illness would progress or what dying would look like.

Eventually, though, the oncology team's cupboard was empty. They referred the couple to an experimental treatment through a clinical trial, which they considered but decided against. Anya vividly recalled that moment they left the cancer center for the last time. "We left the building and every person we had been seeing regularly for two years with no goodbyes, no consultation, no discharge plan, no transition, and no idea what would come next. We felt like our team abandoned us when we needed them the most." Anya and Fred felt they had been "thrown off a cliff."

Consequences: Focusing exclusively on the hopeful road leads to some unfortunate outcomes. Patients and families may not get the full story of their illness trajectory. They're left unprepared when things don't go as hoped, and later on feel misled or betrayed. The doctors and nurses don't know how to move the conversation to the other road of planning. Thus, despite good intentions, important information is withheld, avoided, or sugar-coated. A cone of silence forms between the clinicians and patients.

Susan's Story: In the Know

Just two months after Susan and Geoff celebrated their thirtieth wedding anniversary, Geoff was diagnosed with brain cancer—a high grade glioblastoma. This type of tumor grows extremely quickly and is considered incurable. With surgery and chemotherapy, the average survival time of this type of aggressive brain tumor is fourteen months. Only 5 percent live longer than five years.

Having worked as an occupational therapist for many years, Susan knew they faced a difficult road ahead. Geoff's brain tumor meant he would likely lose language, vision, balance, and personality, depending on where the tumor was located. Susan walked two roads from the very beginning by considering the what-if scenarios. For instance, she obtained medication in case Geoff had a seizure and a medical alert bracelet in case he fell while walking their beloved dog, a bearded collie named Abbie.

During the first year after his diagnosis, Geoff remained stable. Because Susan planned ahead, she wasn't in a panic. She relished this stable phase, which she hoped would last for a long time. Geoff felt well enough to continue walking their dog and spending time with friends and family. In the summer, they traveled with family to his childhood home on the East Coast. He even returned to work.

But Susan knew Geoff's condition would eventually worsen. When treatments no longer worked, he would be discharged from the cancer center. Geoff wanted to die at home. So Susan planned ahead, working with Geoff's family doctor, whom he'd known for several decades, to provide end-of-life care in the home when the time came. This planning reduced the likelihood of unnecessary hospitalizations. In the end, Geoff died peacefully at home surrounded by his family and friends. Because Susan knew the eventual outcome early and the details of how the illness would unfold, she was able to prepare and plan. By the time he passed away, she'd "had a sixteen-month goodbye."

Benefits: Walking two roads is a safeguard against careening from crisis to crisis, especially if you can do so early on. The more information you have—the more realistic, truthful information you can extract from the health care team, other patients, or other resources—the better your experience will be.

How to Walk Two Roads

As Susan and Geoff's story shows, you can remain hopeful even when your illness is incurable and life-limiting. In fact, from the time of diagnosis, patients and families can walk two roads. There are always twists and turns in an illness, so you must be flexible and adjust your hope so it is realistic.

The key Walk Two Roads is fundamentally about making sure you do not get caught up in toxic positivity, a "cross that bridge when we get there" attitude, or an "I would rather not know" mindset. Don't allow these pressures from well-intentioned friends or family, or in the doctor's office, to be barriers to you fully understanding your illness and where you are at in it.

Walk Two Roads is the lynchpin for enacting all the other keys we will explore together. To use this key, you need to be brave. I cannot underscore enough how important it is to ground your whole journey in open, realistic information. I am inviting you to be activated and informed.

Toggle between Planning and Hoping

To walk two roads, you have to allow yourself permission to toggle back and forth between hoping for the best and planning for the rest. In planning mode, you let your mind wander to what-if scenarios and then consider the plan if those should transpire. Some plans might be enacted, some won't be. But giving yourself permission to consider what might happen allows you to seek information for managing those situations should they occur.

Walking two roads is about exploring possibilities but not necessarily having a plan for every single possibility—just the ones that seem most likely. You can make some decisions now and put aside others for later.

The degree to which you focus on one road versus the other will depend. You don't always have to walk each road equally. At times you will feel more optimistic; other times, you'll be more inclined to consider the what-ifs. As with Susan and Geoff, you may find that once you ponder a what-if situation and do some preliminary planning, you can stay on the "hoping for the best" road for longer.

Following major changes in your condition, you may have to make a decision and perhaps quickly—for instance, if you fall. In that case, you can hope to get stronger. But if you don't, you'll want to think about how you will get up and down stairs in your home or what transportation is available. Or when you're moving to or from care settings, say, into the hospital or intensive care unit (ICU), or from these settings or others to home. In these moments, you will want to walk two roads as well. You'll have to keep repeating this process and reassessing your hopes and plans. To do so, you've got to continue to ask your health care providers to describe what might lie ahead and what your options may be.

Walking two roads is a dynamic dance. It is not a one-off exercise. It's something you repeat. It's almost a mindset or philosophy. This requires an element of being brave and resourceful but allows you to be more resilient because you can stay a few steps ahead. Knowing what to expect allows for a greater sense of control over your situation. Again, it's ideal to start toggling back and forth between the two roads early in your illness, so that by the time you're making even bigger decisions, you'll be comfortable doing it.

EXERCISE: HOPE AND PREPARE

It is possible to remain hopeful by adjusting your hopes to match the real situation. You don't need to dwell on the negatives.

Step 1: Fill in the blanks. Based on your situation today, identify things to hope for and to prepare for.

At this stage of your illness journey, what are you hoping for?

1 ____________________

2 ____________________

3 ____________________

4 ____________________

Some examples are:

1. I am hoping that my treatment works.
2. I am hoping that I stay in remission for a long time.
3. I am hoping that I have enough energy to attend my child's graduation or wedding.
4. I am hoping that I can take the vacation I have been planning.

What are the what-if scenarios you are most worried about?

1 ______________________________

2 ______________________________

3 ______________________________

4 ______________________________

Some examples are:

1. What happens if this treatment doesn't work anymore?
2. What happens if I can no longer work?
3. What happens if I cannot drive anymore?
4. What happens if I can no longer care for myself at home?

Step 2: Give yourself permission to let your mind wander. Look at your list of hopes. Toggle back and forth between hoping that those happen and wondering, "What if it doesn't go the way I am hoping?" For the latter, consider what you would need to prepare for or how you might achieve those hopes in a different way. This way of thinking doesn't betray your positive, hopeful vibe. This is a way of remaining real. Balancing hope with the what-ifs.

Step 3: Look at the list of things you are most worried about. Consider what plans you could start exploring sooner rather than later. For example:

1. In case my treatment stops working, I could: create a list of questions for my doctor, make a list of people in my life who will be able to support me, and/or understand what services are available to me.
2. In case I reach a point where I cannot work, I could: talk with a financial advisor and my family about the implications, review ways I can continue to be connected socially, and/or write a list of ways I can create meaning in my life without work.
3. In case I lose my ability to drive, I could: consider how I will remain independent, explore what other modes of transportation are available, ask family or friends to help, and/or research delivery services.
4. In case I cannot care for myself at home, I could: understand options for community in-home services, tour other possible settings of care, and/or discuss the option of moving in with a family member or vice versa.

Step 4: Repeat this exercise as new information or concerns arise, treatments change, or decisions need to be made.

Action 1: Know before You Plan

Knowledge is the foundation of "planning for the rest." Before you can think about the action plan in the event that something goes sideways, you have to know what is likely to happen. Before you can plan for the rest, you must gather accurate information, which you might need to actively seek out because sometimes it's hidden or obscurely presented. The other chapters will help you gather the information you need to be in the know.

Some of that information will lead to planning. Some of it is just important to know and requires no action. But knowing is the key to grounding hope in reality. When you gain factual information, then you can hope accordingly.

When hope is mismatched to the realities of an illness, patients and families get stuck on a path of unrealistic hope. Instead, you want realistic hope. With realistic hope, what you hope for changes as an illness progresses. I've witnessed it over and over in my career: Hope naturally evolves over time when grounded in realistic information. When hope is recalibrated in this way, you have more control and more choices. You can prepare for what is ahead.

Even with a chronic, progressive, life-limiting illness, you can remain hopeful until the very end. You can evolve from hoping for a cure to hoping for stability or a slow disease progression. Over time, you may hope to be cared for, surrounded by those you love, in a place of your preference, such as at home. Hope at the end of life may be less for you and more for your family to be well supported once you pass away.

Cheryl's Story: Evolving Hope

I treated a fifty-five-year-old woman, Cheryl, who had amyotrophic lateral sclerosis (ALS). ALS, also known as Lou Gehrig's disease, is a progressive neurodegenerative disorder. Approximately 80 percent of people with ALS die within two to five years of diagnosis. At the outset and throughout her illness, Cheryl insisted on open conversations with her neurologist about what to expect so that as her situation transitioned, so could her hope.

At first, she hoped that novel treatment options would slow down the progression of her ALS. But despite the medication, over the first year after her diagnosis, she continued to lose the function of her legs. Eventually, she was no longer able to walk. When I first met Cheryl, nearly two years after her diagnosis, she was confined to either her hospital bed or her reclining chair, both in her living room on the main floor. Cheryl hoped that she could remain independent for small tasks like feeding herself or reaching for objects on her bedside table. She also expressed hope that her husband and daughter would be able to work in their careers for as long as possible. She didn't want her illness to derail their lives more than it already had. Now, she hopes that she doesn't choke or suffocate to death, and that when her time comes, she won't linger too long.

I can predict that Cheryl's hope will continue to evolve. As her ALS worsens, she will hope to complete unfinished business or for a visit to the family cottage. Nearing the end, she will hope that she is leaving the world a better place, that her daughter will continue to be a good citizen, that her husband is taken care of and possibly even finds new love. In the end, she will remain as hopeful as she did in the beginning, but the focus of hope will be very different.

Action 2: Role-Model Your Preferred Approach

Walking two roads is a skill that can be done by more than one person. Role modeling how you want to walk your journey, such as openly talking about your desire to walk two roads, will give permission to the people around you to embody this skill as well.

You can invite your inner crew to walk two roads with you. Everyone has an inner crew. It's often made up of those most intimately involved in your illness journey, such as family members, best friends, neighbors, and/or community members. Your inner crew will take the lead from you and likely keep their fears of the what-ifs to themselves. But chances are that everyone is wondering about the same things. When either patients or family members openly talk about walking two roads, everyone will be more able to share the planning and doing together.

To begin communicating your desire to walk two roads, meet with your inner crew one-on-one or in a group. Don't be intimidated to initiate the conversation. You are simply sharing your desire to talk openly about the twists and turns of your illness journey. Often, the members of an inner crew welcome this conversation, as they have been privately wondering the same things as you are. If they are open, you can share with them answers from the exercise earlier in the chapter (on page 35) about your hopes and fears.

Conversation Starters: You can use the following phrases to introduce the skill of walking two roads. Choose the statement that feels most comfortable for you and adapt it however you like:

1 "I appreciate so much that you are in my corner and that you love me. I want to let you know that along this journey, I want to walk two roads, which means hope for the best, and plan for the rest. For me that means..."

2 "I want to have realistic hope throughout my journey. I am asking for your help to be hopeful and realistic at the same time. This will keep me grounded."

3 "I want you to know that it's okay for us to talk openly. It's okay to talk about the hard stuff. For me, that means speaking openly about my illness—for better or for worse—so that I can remain hopeful and prepared at every juncture of my illness."

Don't forget to also tell your health care providers you want to walk two roads. This will make it easier for you to ask about the what-ifs ahead and to seek out realistic information. Doing this can be intimidating. It requires you to be brave and assertive to get the information you need, and willing to hear hard truths. Use versions of the above phrases with them, too, so they understand you want to remain hopeful and prepared at the same time. This will make it easier for them to be open with you.

Family Shout-Out: Sometimes family or inner crew members want to talk openly about the likely scenarios because they have the main responsibility for care and planning, but the patient is hesitant to walk two roads. Here are some example phrases you can use as family or a close friend to explore the patient's willingness to walk two roads:

- "I am in your corner, and I love you so much. I am here for you if you want to walk two roads, which means I will always be hoping for the best, but I will also be here to help you plan for the rest. Is that something you want? And how can I help you do that?"
- "I've read this book and learned how important it is to have realistic hope throughout an illness. The key to realistic hope is walking two roads, which means being hopeful but

also planning for when things go sideways. Walking two roads will increase hope and keep us grounded. How open are you to this idea? What are things you are worried about? What can we prepare for together?"

- "I want you to know that I feel comfortable talking openly about the twists and turns of your illness. I am here to help you prepare if things don't go as hoped. I don't want you to be caught unprepared or to become overwhelmed. Being hopeful and prepared can coexist."

When Someone Doesn't Want to Know

I often get asked what to do if someone in the inner crew doesn't want to know. It's common that someone wants to know more but another doesn't. Sometimes it is the patient who's in denial as the caregiver or family prepares for the future. Other times, the patient wants to prepare for the what-if scenarios, and the family is pressuring them to fight at all costs.

I don't seek to change people's natural styles or personalities. If the patient wants to walk only the road of hope, I will still invite them to know more about their illness and the future. It is important to invite them to the conversation. But I don't force people to engage. I will also invite others, such as the family, by asking whether anyone is interested in learning more about the illness so that they can be prepared if things don't go their way. Sometimes I explore whether it's the family's cultural norm to be more in the know than the patient.

If people are hesitant to talk about the future, they are often scared. I frequently explore their emotions about this rather than provide information. Sometimes I ask what they think about when they let their mind wander, which is an invitation to discuss their worries and fears. Some confide that they are afraid they will fall asleep and never wake up—indicating that they are very aware of dying as a possible outcome but are paralyzed by fear. Others tell me they need to remain stoic to make their families happy, which is an opportunity to debunk the false assumption that hoping for the best is the only and best path.

Sometimes I share the consequences of being in the dark. I tell patients that those who can balance hoping for the best with seeking the truth about the reality of the illness will fare better over time. They'll be more proactive and feel more in control in their illness journey. Again, I'm not forcing them to know the specifics about their illness if they don't want them, but I give them the opportunity to be invited to the conversation.

Lastly, I try to remember that sometimes people need time to absorb information. So, I don't invite people only once. When I visit the next time, I will talk about any changes in their condition, including symptoms or physical decline, and then offer again to talk about what the future might hold. They might take me up on my offer next time. The timing of when they want to be more in the know may change as well. People are ready at different times.

Action 3: Recognize Different Combinations

Ideally, all parties can walk two roads together; however, doing so equally isn't necessary. Some will find it very unsettling to walk two roads. Each family will be different. Not everyone will be able to or want to walk two roads throughout the journey, and this might change at different times.

So that not everyone is going through this journey in the dark, though, someone on the family team—the patient or another member of the inner crew—needs to walk two roads.

Usually, someone will naturally take charge and step into this role. They will need to be brave in seeking realistic information that they may or may not share with the rest of the crew, depending on what each person wants to know.

Tip: Even if someone has chosen to walk only one road, this may change over time. So it may be necessary to keep coming back to this conversation. If others aren't yet able to join you, this should not stop you from seeking out information. Don't be afraid to go solo. For instance, if a patient does not want to walk two roads but their main caregiver does, the caregiver, with permission, could make an appointment alone with the doctors to get the information they need as well as discuss how to manage their own physical and emotional needs.

To illustrate how you can walk two roads at different paces, and how even just one person who walks two roads can help, let me return to the story of Susan and Geoff. As you may remember, Susan began to hope and prepare from the time of Geoff's aggressive brain tumor diagnosis. However, Geoff and his medical team did not.

Geoff wanted as much time as possible. Understandably, he fiercely held on to the hope that he'd do better than the statistics projected. Geoff clung to little signs of hope and avoided dealing with anything related to the inevitable decline. At hospital visits, the health care team members were his great cheerleaders, celebrating what an amazing recovery he had from surgery and how well he was withstanding treatment. He took their cues and was determined to have repeated brain surgeries and live longer.

But during his stable phase, the health care team never explained that it was temporary. Geoff believed he could carry on in a state somewhat close to normal until the one day when death would come. Although his hope was not about being cured, it was stuck in the idea of buying more time. When the doctors told him the cancer was growing, they immediately offered the option of a clinical trial, which involved more experimental chemotherapy. Even though the experimental drug had only a very slim chance of making him live longer, Geoff jumped at the option to sign up for a clinical trial. He received treatment for a few months, until just a few weeks before he died. This decision busied their lives in his final weeks. Had he been able to walk two roads with Susan, he may have chosen to spend his time differently.

Susan learned to walk one road of hope for him, to be optimistic, and walk the other road of preparedness by herself, to prepare for the inevitable changes on her own. She "had to be positive for him," but because she was also proactive and prepared, he was able to die at home, with care from his family doctor, surrounded by his family, friends, and their beloved dog, Abbie.

Kari's Story: Walking Two Roads

To fully illustrate this skill and the practical tips, I want to share a story about Kari, whom I interviewed. She was a caregiver for her daughter, Olivia. Olivia was diagnosed with brain cancer just before her fourteenth birthday. Both mother and daughter, rightfully, were in shock. They'd been planning things like dance lessons and high school courses, and now Olivia needed a brain biopsy and countless tests. With three other children to care for, Kari felt "bombarded" and overwhelmed with anxiety as she worried about the results of the endless stream of tests.

In the beginning, she felt the pressure to stay positive. She was afraid to acknowledge that Olivia could die. "There's the fear inside that if you lose that hope or acknowledge that the person's going to go, it will make them go quicker... Or maybe think, 'it's my fault [if they die], because I didn't hope harder or pray harder,'" she said. But she also realized that she had no power to change cancer. Her daughter's illness was the worst of bad luck. So, she committed to making the best of it.

For Kari, walking two roads came naturally. She is the kind of person who likes to "always prepare for the worst." At the same time, she was "hoping for some kind of miracle" for Olivia. But she realized that she needed to have realistic hope and be prepared if she wanted to make the most of the time Olivia had left.

But it wasn't just Kari who walked two roads. Olivia did as well. Olivia was also role modeling for her mother and family how to be hopeful and realistic. In a way, Olivia set the stage for her family members, and they followed her lead. Olivia was "aware of everything and nothing was kept from her" regarding her disease progression. The doctors were straight with her. But she didn't dwell on the negative. Instead, she had as much fun, love, and affection as she could during the time she had.

As Olivia's illness progressed, she handled it with grace and dignity, hope and preparedness. On one hand, Olivia expressed to her mother that she didn't want to keep living if her whole life was going to be in a state of suffering. On the other hand, she recalibrated her hopes at each major change in her condition. She still ardently followed her dreams and pursued her plans. She continued going to school, in a wheelchair. Her mom transported her from the car to the wheelchair so she could take private classes. Kari said, "She was living each day. Right to the end, we had teachers come to the house with her sitting in her wheelchair. She couldn't walk, but she still wanted to learn as much as she could."

Olivia and Kari experienced hope evolving over time. The hope at the beginning was that the treatments would shrink the tumor so it could be operated on. Unfortunately, the tumor did not shrink. Then they began to hope that another treatment could be done. When no new treatments were available, they hoped the tumor would not grow quickly. Whenever they learned that the tumor was growing, Kari kept hoping that Olivia would remain "stable, in that spot, for as long as possible." They found ways to make her comfortable. They kept hoping that she would be able to have some quality of life and enjoy the time she had left.

Kari and Olivia's journey was not a straight line. They continually toggled back and forth between hoping for the best and planning for the rest, sometimes planning how to arrange her schooling or physiotherapy, other times hoping a treatment was going to give Olivia more time. The road was unpredictable. Kari said that the split between being hopeful and being prepared is never fifty-fifty. "You're always going to waver and go back and forth. It's more like a curve. Actually, it's just like a roller coaster," she said.

Even though Olivia and Kari walked two roads, not everyone in their family did. Olivia's father could not accept that there was going to be an end to Olivia's life. He spent all this time trying to find a cure. He would desperately take Olivia and Kari to various appointments across town, trying all kinds of alternative remedies. Kari said, "I worry he really lost out on his time with Olivia. And I feel sad for that."

Ultimately, the benefit of walking two roads throughout was that it helped Kari and Olivia have a close and loving relationship. During this incredibly stressful time, they strengthened their bond. Kari said, "The ability to walk two roads allowed me to really be there for Olivia, in every way. It drew us closer. We became inseparable best friends."

Olivia died about two years after her diagnosis, at age sixteen. Kari, though heartbroken, did not bear guilt or regret when her daughter died. She felt at peace, knowing she did everything she could in the way Olivia wanted. In walking two roads, she was able to enjoy the precious time she had with her daughter, grounded in realistic hope.

Walk Two Roads: Summary

- Hope for the best and plan for the rest. Planning does not betray hope. Hope naturally evolves, but only if you have information about the truth of your illness.
- Toggle between being hopeful and being realistic and prepared for how the story might unfold.
- Walk two roads as early as you can; it will prevent you from feeling blindsided later. As your journey unfolds, check in to obtain information about whether your illness is changing so you can recalibrate hope to reality if necessary.

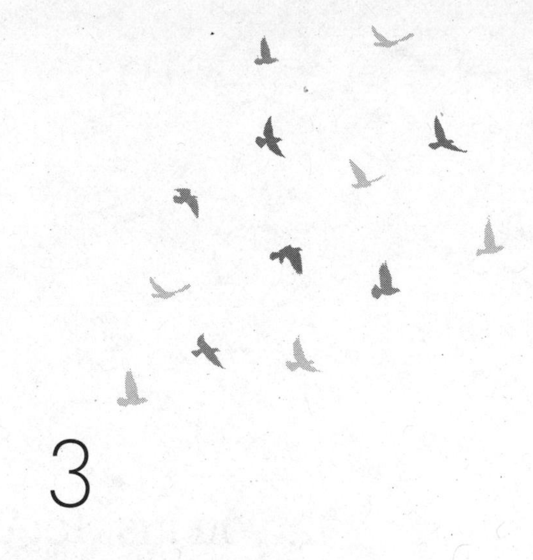

3

ZOOM OUT

“If you just focus on the smallest details, you will never get the big picture right.”

LEROY HOOD

THE KEY Zoom Out means being able to step back and understand the overall storyline of an illness and where you are within it. It is about knowing the bird's-eye view of your specific serious illness, which serves as a road map for you.

Assumption: The Future Is Unknown

Most people assume there is no crystal ball to predict the future. Sometimes clinicians say that exact phrase to patients, by which they mean, "No one knows how this disease will unfold for you exactly." Every patient is different, after all.

There is uncertainty with any life-changing diagnosis. So many factors can vary immensely: the disease itself, how it presents, how effective treatment will be, what new treatments might be available in the future, and so on. But patients are looking for what to expect. At some point in their illness, they may ask questions like, "What happens next?" "What happens if this treatment doesn't work?" Depending on the illness, in an attempt to understand how serious it is, they might even ask, "How much time do I have?"

Many clinicians and providers are uncomfortable with uncertainty. Because they want to be cheerful and optimistic, they give vague answers. They will say things like, "Let's cross that bridge when we get there" or "Let's take things one day at a time." Some might even deflect the question by saying another doctor should answer it. All of this leaves patients and families incorrectly assuming that the future is completely unknown.

Reality: Every Serious Illness Has a Pattern

The reality is that every serious illness follows a general pattern, often referred to as the "natural history" of the disease. It's the long-range forecast of the illness based on the patterns of the millions of people who have had the disease before. This natural history does not predict exactly each individual's experience through the illness, but it can provide patients and families with a road map of what the average journey looks like.

Common diseases have a typical progression. Health care providers can recognize each of the stages of an illness because they have treated many other patients with those diseases. When it cannot be cured, cancer has a general pattern, as do heart failure and end-stage lung disease, Parkinson's disease, dementia, ALS, frailty, and so on. Each illness pattern is different.

Generally speaking, every illness, just like every story, has beginning, middle, late, and end chapters. These chapters might be short or long, depending on the story. These chapters have milestones and decision points that are well known by clinicians. Patients should expect these along the way. Knowing about them can help you predict the rhythm and cadence of the illness over time.

Elizabeth's Story: In the Dark

I met a sixty-three-year-old woman named Elizabeth, whom for many years had two diseases affecting her lungs and heart: chronic obstructive pulmonary disease (COPD) and congestive heart failure. She'd been admitted to the hospital almost monthly over eight months with a flare-up of one or both illnesses. She'd never spent more than two weeks at home between visits. Everyone in the hospital knew her by her first name. Each flare-up started the same way: she'd develop a hacking cough, breathlessness, and swollen legs. She and her husband would wait it out anxiously for a few days because she was tired of hospitals, but the symptoms would persist. Her husband would eventually take her to the emergency department and she would be hospitalized. In the hospital, staff would treat the immediate issue, such as a pneumonia. Once she was stable, she would be sent home.

She was taking things one day at a time. But the vicious cycle continued. No one explained to her that they could not fix the underlying conditions and that her serious illnesses were progressing. She didn't realize that each episode chipped away at her baseline, and she never fully bounced back to where she'd been before the last admission. These symptoms weren't one-off issues but were likely to recur and worsen. Had she had a sense of the bigger picture of her illness, she might have worked with her health care team to plan to avoid going to the hospital yet still be comfortable.

Consequences: Without the information about what to expect next, patients make uninformed decisions. Patients and families feel caught in a vortex, confused as to where the path will lead, looking only at what's in front of them and living in the day-to-day. They are missing the bird's-eye view of where they are in their illness.

Carla's Story: In the Know

I'll give you an example of how information about an illness' storyline can be powerful. I have a physician colleague who works in neuro-oncology and also practices zooming out. He says that decisions for any treatment, especially for someone with a progressive, life-limiting illness, need to be made with a realistic understanding of the person's prognosis. His patient Carla had a devastating brain cancer that is typically treated with surgery, if possible, followed by chemotherapy and radiation. After these treatments, patients essentially wait for their disease to recur.

Carla had all the treatments. She was stable for a time, and then her cancer recurred. Over a couple of weeks of clinic visits, she showed significant decline in her function. My colleague discussed giving her a course of steroids, which decreases swelling in the brain but always temporarily. He explained to Carla and her family that the steroids were not a cure. They would make symptoms better, sometimes significantly, but eventually the symptoms would return. Once symptoms come back, steroids have much less of an effect. It was a one-time treatment option. Carla understood this and decided to take the steroid prescription. Two weeks later, when he met Carla again in the clinic, she told him that she had improved significantly. She'd had an incredible two weeks with visits from family from across the country. She wouldn't trade that time for anything. But now, some of the symptoms had started to come back and she was struggling with the side effects of the steroids. But she'd had a tremendous two weeks with new, meaningful memories with her family. Everyone knew this was the last time that she'd be able to improve before getting worse. They were extremely thankful for this time.

Benefits: By putting things in context, Carla and her family could take advantage of a two-week window. Carla zoomed in by taking the treatment for her swelling, which helped her feel better. She zoomed out by seeing and accepting this as a temporary measure given that she was progressing through her illness. She understood the bird's-eye view. This allowed her and her family to plan better and treasure spending quality time together.

How to Zoom Out

Upon receiving a diagnosis of a serious illness, you usually get very busy. Treatment plans are discussed and often chosen. You scramble to keep up with the day-to-day issues related to the illness—the tests, appointments, procedures, side effects, and so on. Each visit is focused on the blood test results, the latest scan, the most pressing symptom, the immediate next step.

I call this zooming in. It is much easier for health care providers to focus on the day-to-day issue rather than talk about the big picture. It's like they are busy focusing on the hourly weather of the illness instead of stepping back to describe the long-range forecast with you. But when the big picture is lost, so are you.

There will be times during your illness when you'll want to zoom in, and other times when you will need to zoom out. But during major transition points, you'll need to do both. Some of these transition points include when an unexpected complication requires a sudden decision, when you are moving across care settings, when you change treatments, or when you notice a decline in your physical function or stamina. When these occur, the big picture needs to be revisited, reinforced, and recontextualized.

I find that too often, patients stay zoomed in, getting lost in the weeds of their illness. Without a big-picture context, you can be caught in a chaotic rhythm that feels like one crisis after another. There is no opportunity to step back and prepare for the next curveball of an illness. You may become trapped in a reactive state, always caught off guard, and miss the telltale signs that speak to the illness' progression.

To zoom out properly, you need to do two things: get a bird's-eye view of the illness and future gaze.

Bird's-Eye View

When I meet my patients, one of the first things I do is ask them what has happened since the diagnosis and what is their understanding of where things are at with their illness. I then offer to share the natural history of their illness. Understanding the natural phases of an illness and which phase you are in will give you context and help you anticipate what lies ahead in your life.

Imagine you're in an outdoor garden maze with very high hedges. From within the maze, you lack perspective. At the ground level, you don't know if you should turn right or left or what turn will lead to a dead end. But if you were to look down at the maze from a bird's-eye view, you would see the pathway. In the same way, zooming out shows you where you are in your illness so that you can choose the next right step for the quality of life you want to live.

Conversation Starters: Here are ways to ask your health care provider about the bird's-eye view of your illness:

- "Please help me understand the big picture or average journey of this illness."
- "Can you help me get a bird's-eye view of where I am in this illness journey now?"
- "Am I in the beginning, middle, late, or end stage of this illness?"
- "Am I in the first half or the second half of my illness?"

Future Gazing

With the context of a bird's-eye view of their illness, I often invite my patients to time travel with me. I ask them whether they ever wonder about the future. And I ask their permission to imagine together what the future will look like. I often share that I have cared for many people with similar illnesses, and I have information about what the future may look like. And if they want to know, we can explore together.

They almost always take me up on my invitation. When they do, I help them walk the road of planning for the rest. In fact, I often explore multiple roads, and toggle back and forth between potential scenarios. This allows them to be more in the know and in control.

If they are hesitant, I do not force them to explore the future. But I do try to dispel the myth that knowing more will lead to feeling depressed. In my experience, people don't feel hopeless or fearful when they receive factual and meaningful information. They feel more grounded. It may take a few moments for them to swallow the fact that the illness is going to follow a particular pattern. But people typically adjust. And they use this information as power.

The power comes from having the opportunity to plan ahead—they can predict the scenarios that are likely to occur and stay one step ahead of the illness. They know what to expect as a normal part of their illness and have realistic hope. This information is empowering because patients and families can make decisions that are best for them in the context of the estimated time they have left. No one else can make those decisions as knowledgeably as they can.

Conversation Starters: Here are ways you can ask your health care providers about future gazing:

- "What can I expect in the next stages of my illness?"
- "What will my illness look like moving forward?"
- "What major hurdles or challenges should I expect along the way?"
- "What big decisions will I face in the future?"

Action 1: Visualize the Illness Trajectory

Patients tend to find it helpful when I draw their illness trajectory on a piece of paper. An illness trajectory shows the pattern of physical decline for that illness by plotting the physical functioning or stamina over time. With this, patients and families can visualize the overall storyline, where they are now, and where they might be headed. Sometimes a patient thinks they are in the early stage of a disease and the health care provider thinks they are in the middle to late stage. Visualizing the illness trajectory promotes a clearer understanding for all sides.

Dr. Joanne Lynn, geriatrician and health services researcher, and her colleagues first published about illness trajectories as a way to describe how each illness has a different rhythm and pattern to it, which should inform care priorities. I'll explain the most common illness trajectories, but before I do, please note that the illness trajectories represent general patterns. Not everyone with cancer has a short period of steady decline, for instance. But many have some version of this. So it still is possible to describe the average pattern for every illness, even though everyone is different.

For those dying from a car accident, a sudden heart attack, or suicide, their physical function is high over time, and then there is a sudden straight drop downward at the moment of death (see figure 1).

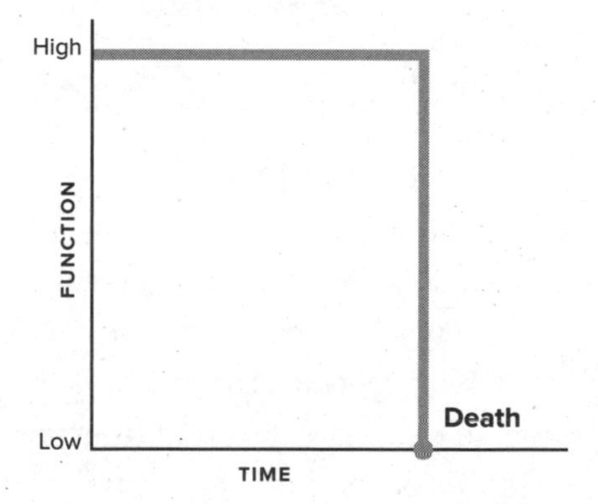

FIGURE 1.
Illness trajectory typical of traumatic event or accident

Patients with diseases like advanced cancer have a substantial period of high function followed by a period of steady decline (see figure 2). There comes a point at which the illness overwhelms the patient's function, and stamina usually declines quite steadily in the final months and weeks before death.

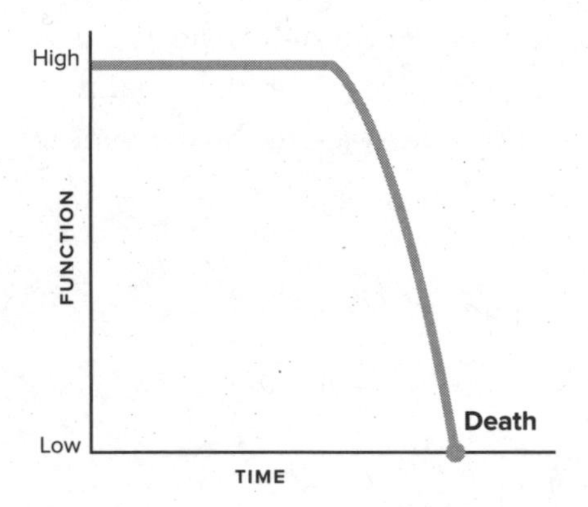

FIGURE 2.
Illness trajectory typical of non-curable cancer

The trajectory of long decline with intermittent episodes is characterized by erratic exacerbations causing periods of sudden decline with a backdrop of overall gradual decline. Patients with major organ system failure, such as congestive heart failure or COPD, typically live for a relatively long time with their illness, with minor limitations in everyday life. From time to time, they experience a worsening of serious symptoms or a stress that overwhelms the body's reserves (for example, pneumonia or a heart attack), which often leads to hospitalization. Patients recover from such episodes but never quite regain the same function as before (see figure 3). Their pattern is marked by these intermittent serious exacerbations over time, until they experience an episode or complication from which they cannot recover.

Trajectory of Long Decline with Intermittent Episodes

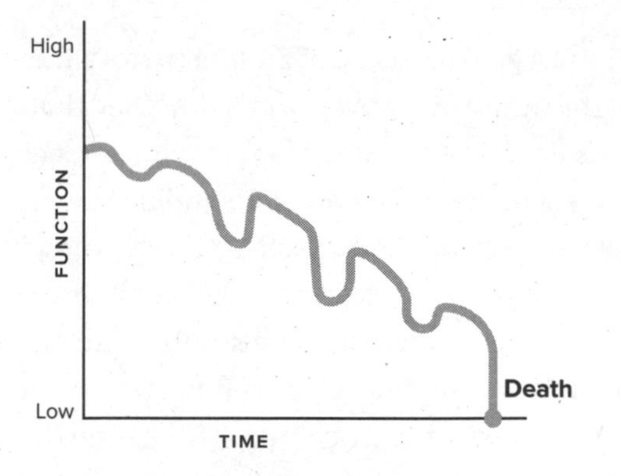

FIGURE 3.
Illness trajectory typical of major organ system failure, such as heart failure

The trajectory of prolonged dwindling is characterized by low, gradual decline. Patients with neurological failures (such as Alzheimer's disease or other forms of dementia) or general frailty of multiple body systems are typically older. They often have low to very low function for a prolonged time, sometimes years and years (see figure 4). Changes can be subtle. The support services required can be intense, such as needing institutional long-term care facilities.

Trajectory of Prolonged Dwindling

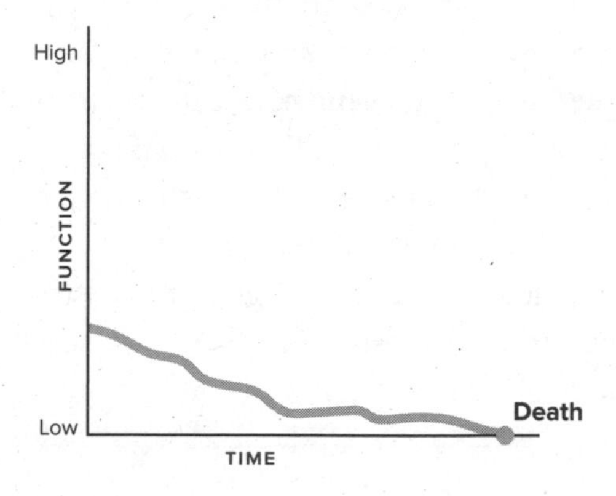

FIGURE 4.
Illness trajectory typical of dementia, disabling stroke, or frailty

Action 2: Learn the "Story" of the Illness

Drawing it out gives you a general sense of an illness storyline, specifically the physical decline; however, you need other vital information about the details of the story to fully understand the milestones you'll encounter, what a change might mean, and how it will impact day-to-day aspects of your life. Knowing the details will also equip you to understand whether there are new decisions to be made or what-if scenarios to consider.

Below, I present a generic, high-level storyline of what to expect in the different stages of the three major-illness trajectories. This is an example of the type of details you can expect and ask for from your clinical team. I leave the details of how to know if you are moving from the late stage of a life-limiting illness (for example, the last year of life) to the end stage (for example, the last weeks of life) for later in the book, for if and when you want more information.

Story of Steady Decline

In the beginning, patients who have an illness such as a non-curable cancer will often remain reasonably "hearty" for some time after diagnosis. From a functional perspective (referring to overall physical stamina), some may have a period of stability that lasts for years. During this time, they might receive a variety of cancer-related treatments, or surgery, which may cause different side effects, or they might face intermittent acute issues like infection or fever. Generally, each time these acute issues are treated, patients bounce back to their baseline stamina. The overall trend of stability continues.

Inevitably, in the middle stages of this trajectory, a patient's body begins to decline. They don't respond as well to the treatments as they previously did. Some switch to a new treatment regimen, which may be effective or maintain the steady state so the cancer is neither shrinking nor growing.

Eventually, in the late stage, a patient typically loses their appetite but often feels the need to encourage themselves to eat. They might lose weight. They start feeling more tired. They seem to fatigue more easily, so they naturally pace themselves during activity. They may not walk as far or go out as much. Getting to appointments is more taxing and tiring. They start to take more naps. If they run into acute issues like an infection, instead of bouncing back after treatment like they did before, the trend continues downward without returning to the previous baseline. They seem to be "running out of gas."

Story of Long Decline with Intermittent Episodes

In the beginning, after an organ failure diagnosis, the initial goal is to maximize the functioning of that failing organ (heart, lung, kidney, etc.). Chronic, progressive, or life-limiting organ illnesses are marked with episodes of acute exacerbations along the patient's journey. These happen intermittently and erratically.

Episodes are characterized by sudden, severe worsening of symptoms typically requiring immediate medical attention, most commonly in the hospital setting and sometimes the ICU. For example, patients with COPD can experience sudden shortness of breath over a few days with a worsening productive cough and a general feeling of being unwell. If left unattended, the episode can quickly escalate to an emergency situation where the patient might have to be temporarily put on breathing machines. These episodes are usually related to a chest infection causing pneumonia; so, antibiotics are usually ordered while the breathing is stabilized. Acute setbacks like this frighten patients but often they pull through and are discharged home.

In the middle stage, what is often missed in this illness pattern is that patients don't quite ever get back to their baseline heartiness after an exacerbation, because each episode has taken a toll. But because they survived, their recovery is celebrated and the subtle decline between episodes is overlooked. Over a period of time, these patients will begin a downward trend.

In the late stage, this decline is similar to that described in the previous illness trajectory. Patients with end organ failure start to exhibit more fatigue, weakness, low stamina, and energy. They lose their appetite and overall heartiness. They begin a functional decline, needing more assistance, and eventually become more homebound. Gradually, the general steady decline is more prominent than the exacerbations. This is when it is obvious that further hospitalizations won't prolong the patient's life, even when there is another exacerbation. The focus remains on comfort and supportive care throughout.

Story of Prolonged Dwindling

At the beginning of this illness trajectory, the patient population, such as those with dementia or frailty, has an extremely gradual functional decline that usually occurs over many years, even a decade. When changes to stamina and heartiness happen at a snail's pace, sometimes it isn't noticed.

In the middle stage, people generally struggle with stamina, and they will exhibit a decline over time. Their walking slows, their ability to get up from a chair becomes strained, and they increasingly become weaker. They might have weight loss because of poor appetite. They sleep for increasingly longer periods. Eventually, they become more homebound. Mobility aids are increasingly needed to get around. Fortunately, this illness trajectory isn't plagued with exacerbations or high symptom burdens. Thus, background functional decline is similar to the first two illness trajectories; it just seems like more of a marathon.

During the late stage, the speed at which the decline in stamina is happening predicts the person's timeline. Year to year, month to month, week to week, or day to day—trends are more telling than the odd bad day.

EXERCISE: LEARN THE STORYLINE

Ask your clinician to draw the storyline or trajectory of your illness on a piece of paper. Visuals can reinforce what the overarching pattern will look like. You can even ask your clinician to mark the spot where they think you are in the trajectory.

Even with these generic storylines, you still have to customize them to your illness and situation. Ask your clinician if your understanding of the storyline is correct. Find out:

- What signs will indicate what stage you are in
- What to expect from each stage
- What will be the decision points along the way
- What are the important things to do in each stage of your illness

Revisit the storyline with your clinician over time, especially whenever there are major changes in the illness. Major events like falls, hospitalizations, or a large loss of function are all triggers to revisit the big picture of the illness and ask questions. Contextualizing these changes along the trajectory will help you figure out where you're at and what's coming ahead. You can also ask your health care provider how often you should revisit this discussion.

Using the Storyline to Your Advantage

Once you and your clinician have filled in the narrative around the beginning, middle, and late chapters of your illness, it is important to understand how the storyline will affect your life. This means considering how the expected physical changes at each stage might impact your everyday life. Take for example an illness like ALS. This is an illness with a known progression, with well-described stages and turning points. People with ALS may lose their fine motor skills and find it difficult to write. They will lose the ability to swallow and possibly speak.

So a person with early-stage ALS might think about what they most want to communicate and with whom when they are not able to speak and write. They might want to write letters or record messages for their loved ones while they are still able. They might explore options for creative communication modalities so they can maintain their "voice" in some way down the road. For instance, world-famous physicist Stephen Hawking had an unusual course of ALS, which over decades paralyzed him; but his mind was still sharp and he communicated through a speech-generating device initially controlled by his hands and eventually by his cheek muscles.

At some point, since mobility is going to become a challenge, patients might want to start exploring modifications to their home, like ramps or a walk-in bathtub. They could explore mobility aids and technologies like wheelchairs or lifts. They might start exercises to preserve their strength for longer. Similarly, since swallowing will become a challenge, they may want to make their wishes known with regard to a feeding tube.

Another example is a patient with dementia. If a person knows that at some point their memory is going to worsen, they might want to take the time beforehand to get their affairs in order. For instance, while they are still cognitively well enough to understand and consent, they should attend to important legal and financial matters, such as picking a health care proxy or substitute decision maker and sharing their values and preferences.

Knowing what is likely to happen in the future stages of an illness affects how you live your life and your overall quality of life. Try to foresee and prepare for decisions that may need to be made. There are many practical things to address. But there are also emotional, social, and financial implications. These are best not done in a crisis. Knowing the trajectory and details is not enough. To stay more grounded and in control, go one level deeper and consider all the implications. This is how you stay two steps ahead of your illness.

Action 3: Separate the Storyline from the Timeline

Zooming out to understand the overarching road map is not the same thing as asking how long you will stay in this stage of an illness or how much time you have left. The big-picture storyline of the illness is well known, but the timing can vary from person to person. Mapping the timelines of a typical storyline is a bit like mapping the timelines of puberty. We know generally what is going to happen during puberty, such as hormonal changes, voice changes, and body hair growth. But the timing varies from person to person. Some people blossom early, some later. Every individual experiences puberty differently, but the pattern is well known.

Some patients with life-limiting conditions may want to know how the illness will affect their lifespan. When people google their disease or speak with their doctor, they may learn about the average survival time. This is the average time from diagnosis to death based on millions of people who have had the same illness. Of course, some people live longer and some shorter than the average. Yet I find that many people fixate on the average survival time, thinking of it like a countdown or expiry date.

The table below shows the average population timelines for some of the more common chronic, progressive, and life-limiting illnesses from the time of diagnosis.

Average Timelines for Chronic, Progressive, and Life-Limiting Illnesses

Dementia or Alzheimer's disease	5–15 years
Congestive heart failure (CHF)	5–15 years
Chronic obstructive pulmonary disease (COPD)	10–15 years
Pulmonary fibrosis (PF)	3–6 years
Cystic fibrosis (CF)	44 years (total lifespan)
Cirrhosis	10–15 years
Chronic kidney disease (CKD)	20–40 years
Amyotrophic lateral sclerosis (ALS)	2–5 years
Progressive supranuclear palsy	6–10 years
Multiple system atrophy	8–12 years
Parkinson's disease	10–15 years
Non-curable cancers	Varies greatly by type of cancer
Frailty condition or syndrome	Variable

However, within each illness, there are different sub-types of illness and there is a great deal of variability depending on different factors. This is why many doctors hesitate to answer questions about prognosis. They know there is variation with the average survival time; they don't want to over- or underestimate the time left for you individually. It is easy to accurately predict survival time in a large population but hard to do so accurately at an individual level, especially early on in an illness.

Understanding the stages you will go through and what to look for when you're approaching the middle and later part of an illness will be important to your quality of life and ability to make future decisions. Nonetheless, the stages you'll go through are distinct from the average survival time. I have found that once people understand the difference between storyline and timeline, most want to know about the storyline but not all want to know about the average timeline. Whether you want to know only one or the other, or both, all options are okay.

Information about the average timeline of most illnesses is readily available on the Internet, but information about the narrative storyline of the illness is hard to find. Existing educational materials, while helpful, tend to focus on the biomedical and physiological aspects of the illness. The information often lacks practical details of how biological changes will affect your quality of life and the important decisions you might have to face at each stage.

Conversation Starters: If you are interested in the average timeline of your illness, you can ask the following:

- "Can you help me understand the average timeline for someone with this illness?"
- "How long do people typically live with this illness?"
- "What is the average prognosis for someone with this illness?"

If a health care provider responds with a version of "I don't have a crystal ball," you can follow up with, "I know you cannot predict survival time to an exact science. But what is the average timeline or range that one can expect, based on your own experience or the natural history of the disease?"

Daren's Story: Zooming Out

Dr. Daren Heyland is a professor of medicine and epidemiology at Queen's University in Ontario, Canada, and a critical-care doctor working in the ICU. He is also a health care researcher focused on improving communication and decision-making for very sick patients facing serious illnesses.

He told me that the idea of zooming out resonated strongly with him in his work as an ICU doctor caring for very sick patients on a daily basis. Health care providers "are too often in the weeds," he said, "talking about details of different treatments as if they're on a menu. Do you want CPR? With or without intubation? With or without a defibrillator? It just breaks [these decisions] down into these little pieces. And what is more helpful is to back up out of the weeds, zoom out, and really understand what should be governing these decisions."

Dr. Heyland shared an anecdote about a heart-wrenching bereavement interview he conducted as part of one of his research studies. The study followed patients with advanced disease and their caregivers over time, interviewed them to understand their unmet needs, and then intervened with tailored solutions. An older person with metastatic prostate cancer was recruited into the study and he subsequently passed away. A month after he died, Dr. Heyland conducted the interview with the man's wife.

This older couple had been facing a well-documented, chronic, life-limiting illness. They'd been interacting with the health system, likely for several years. In the couple's last visit with their medical team before the man died, the medical team talked about the patient's PSA (prostate specific antigen) levels, but no one explained to the couple what those rising levels meant or let them know that time was running short. The wife didn't have a sense that the end of her husband's life was near, and she missed out on being able to say goodbye and have closure to a forty-year marriage.

Dr. Heyland has also used the key of zooming out in planning with his own family. He told me he'd moved back to his hometown in Alberta to be closer to his aging parents. He soon realized something was wrong with his mother. He suspected dementia, which was later confirmed. Because he had insider knowledge of the trajectory of dementia, he could coach his family, particularly his father, through a transition from denial to grief to acceptance. "My father and my sisters, in particular, needed that kind of coaching to appreciate the bigger picture," Dr. Heyland told me.

He and I talked about the "dance" that occurs between zooming in and zooming out over an illness. His siblings had grabbed at possible cures, treatments, and complementary medicines for their mother to try to slow her decline. That strategy had value in small doses, he said, "but what happens too often is people just stay zoomed in. And if that's the only strategy, you're going to miss opportunities for important conversations, [which] eventually my mother lost the capacity to have."

One of the messages in this chapter is that once you have a sense of the overarching pattern, you can revisit where you are in it to inform your decisions. Dr. Heyland talked about this in the context of caring for his mother. He was grateful that the family had relished the time they had with her—that they had said what they needed to say while she was alert and present. His entire extended family had even gone to Hawaii and spent a week at the beach with his mom and dad. His mother is from South Africa and "being on the ocean was so meaningful," Dr. Heyland told me. "To have her feet washed by the waves and the sound of the ocean" meant the world to him and his family. "That was three years ago. Now, none of that could happen given where her disease is at."

Ultimately, knowing the big picture has helped him and his family manage his mom's advanced dementia. He summarized the benefit of zooming out: "We are constantly looking at the big picture, trying to anticipate what's going to happen next. 'What's the next requirement going to be? Who do I need to mobilize to meet that care need?' Whereas if you're focused on the here and now, and only zoomed in, you'll be caught off guard and you'll always be catching up. Zooming out allows us to be sure that we're attending to what's important to this person on their life journey, given that bigger picture."

Zoom Out: Summary

- Every life-changing illness has a natural history or illness trajectory to it. This information can ground you by providing a bird's-eye view of what to expect along the journey.
- Most health care providers are not trained in talking about the big picture of an illness. Instead, they are zoomed in on the latest scan or blood test or acute symptom and the like.
- Ask about the illness trajectory and details of the storyline early so you can use this information to check in throughout the illness. This information can serve as a road map for the right decisions for you and to anticipate potential changes over time.

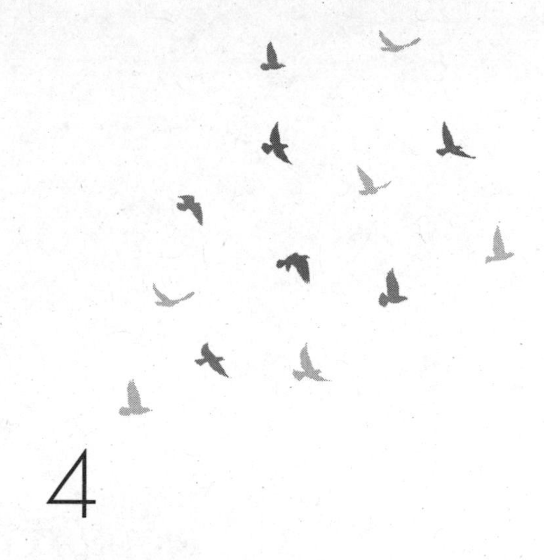

4

KNOW YOUR STYLE

“A leopard never changes its spots.”

DERIVED FROM JEREMIAH 13:23

THE KEY Know Your Style means harnessing your awareness of your personal style and how you deal with challenges. There are positive and negative aspects to everyone's style, and these usually become amplified over the course of an illness. Harnessing this information will enable you to gain more control of your illness story.

Assumption: The Disease Is the Full Story

Most people assume their illness experience is driven entirely by what happens with the disease. Their attention is focused on the diagnosis, how bad it is, what bodily organs it has affected, how much it has changed between medical appointments, and so on. They spend their time and energy researching the treatments available. Some travel great distances to access the best doctors and hospitals.

There are no guarantees in medicine, so at some point, there is uncertainty about how an illness will respond to treatment or how it will unfold, especially for non-curable illnesses. Thus, because in many ways patients cannot control what happens with the illness, they feel as if they are losing control of their life. I've had patients say to me, "I reoriented my life around the illness."

Reality: Your Style Will Greatly Influence the Story

Focusing mainly on the illness isn't wrong, but it is an incomplete view. Intrinsically, you have important information that can predict how you will walk through this journey. There are patterns in your life. How a person has dealt with challenges in their past holds important clues about how they will manage a serious illness in the future. For instance, how they handled divorce, breakups, or adversity. Similarly, how they interact with family and friends can be predictive of how they will engage with the health care system.

You have inherent skills and traits that have brought you to where you are today. You need to be aware of those skills so you can leverage them to make your experience more positive. This can increase your hopefulness because you're reviewing the ways you have been resilient in the face of challenges throughout your life. It can also be a moment of reflection to identify strategies that didn't work well and need modification or support to change.

This idea of one's style influencing the illness journey can arise in many ways. Here are some common examples of the consequences of neglecting people's natural styles:

- A wife gets frustrated that her partner is not interested in joining her in the room for the doctor visits, even though the partner has avoided bad news their whole life and finds dealing with sad news traumatic.

- A single father's condition is deteriorating and he requires more help to move around. The son, who lives with the father, is frustrated that his sister never comes around to help out, even though she usually visits only twice a year, on holidays.
- A man has always been indecisive, needing ample time to consider options before making any decision. He gets sick and is offered several treatment options. His wife is frustrated and angry that he can't make a timely decision on such an important matter.
- A woman complains that her older sister insists on attending every appointment with her, shows up at the house often, and won't give her any space or privacy. Yet the older sister has always been the kind of person who seeks a lot of information, has always been very protective of her little sister, and shows her love by doing tasks.

The Bickersons' Story: In the Dark

I cared for a couple who had an acrimonious, volatile, and dysfunctional marriage. Let's call them Mr. and Mrs. Bickerson. The Bickersons did not get along throughout their entire marriage, but they stayed together. They never could see eye to eye. When Mrs. Bickerson developed a progressive illness, Mr. Bickerson became her caregiver. But that was a completely unnatural relationship for them to be in.

She continued to feel that he never did enough for her, that he didn't really care for her, and that he wanted her to die quickly. She told him repeatedly that he was just a nuisance, that there was nothing he could do right for her, and that she had no faith in him as a caregiver. He felt unappreciated, badgered, belittled, and emasculated. I tried to support them along with a spiritual counselor I work with. We identified that these were long-standing themes in their relationship. Neither of them was about to change, especially during a more heightened emotional crisis. One could have anticipated their issues would be amplified during the illness. They had never been able to negotiate or console or care for each other. It was a doomed setup from the start. Had they appreciated that, they may not have entered into the relationship of patient and caregiver.

Consequences. The Bickersons suffered. Not appreciating their own styles and how this could affect the illness story amplified the suffering. Had they been more aware, perhaps they would have hired someone or involved another family member. Only fixating on an illness and not appreciating how a person's style can affect the illness experience can lead people to more suffering, and to feeling unsure, helpless, and powerless.

Rosalie's Story: In the Know

To illustrate how knowing your style can affect your experience, I want to tell the story of Rosalie. Rosalie is a seventy-eight-year-old caregiver to her husband, Paul, whom she calls her "prince." They've been married for fifty-nine years. Paul was diagnosed with pancreatic cancer over three years ago.

When reflecting on her style, Rosalie describes herself as a full-fledged "mama bear"—ready to protect her husband and kids from everything. She's the kind of person who likes to prepare herself for every situation, so she is ready to act when something needs to be done. When she herself was diagnosed with breast cancer, she researched and then insisted on a mastectomy. When the surgeon wanted to offer her other options, she said loudly: "You're not listening to me! I want my breast removed. That is what I want." Her husband, however, is "the opposite." He doesn't really like talking much about problems when they arise. He likes to look "on the bright side" and avoids talking about negative things.

By reflecting on his style compared to hers, she could approach him with more understanding. "We both attack this in different ways because we're different people," she told me. By thinking about their differing styles, she became "more aware of what he's like," and encouraged a different dialogue between them. Rosalie recognized that Paul needed more time to adjust to changes in routine than she did. Plus, he didn't like to dwell on negative things.

When they met with the oncologist, she wanted Paul to ask a question about the timeline of his illness. But "he absolutely flew off the handle." He wasn't ready. She reiterated that he was in charge; they were his questions to ask. She also knew she could make her own appointment with the oncologist to ask questions directly. So she pulled back and gave him space. His style wasn't to be so direct. But later on, he asked Rosalie whether he was in remission or not. She suggested asking the doctor this, and that began a discussion with the medical team about his illness storyline. Without appreciating that he needed to ask on his terms, Rosalie, with her "mama bear" style, might have closed Paul off completely to the questions.

Knowing her style helped Rosalie understand her husband and how he needs to handle his illness better, and vice versa. Paul and Rosalie could have knocked heads if they hadn't appreciated their respective styles. They might have misinterpreted each other. He might have thought she was being pushy;

she might have thought he was keeping her in the dark. Instead, Rosalie appreciated that they offer each other different things. As a result, Rosalie felt seen. She told me: "It validated the way I deal with my husband. It validated who I am as a caregiver. I was on the right track."

Benefits. The personality and individual style of patients and families can predict how they will conduct themselves through the illness, for better or worse. Know Your Style is the antidote to feelings of helplessness. This information can ground you and is not tied to any test result. It is a way to gain some control over how you will journey through this illness. Ultimately, you can use this knowledge to identify things that help and hinder the illness journey and implement strategies to prepare.

How to Know Your Style

As a doctor, I spend a lot of time asking people about who they are as a person. I ask about how they have lived, especially when they have faced other challenges, such as a divorce, a job loss, or a death in the family. How did they react? What were their coping mechanisms? What were their tendencies? This also involves taking stock of a person's style of information seeking. This is all important knowledge that can predict how someone will manage the illness experience as much as the illness itself.

To know your style means to reflect on your personality, tendencies, and strategies when you faced challenges in the past. It is important to do this whether you are the patient or in the inner crew.

Knowing your style, you can proactively implement strategies to manage the uncertainties ahead and the ebbs and flows of the disease. This is important because there are limits to your ability to change the disease, but you can take charge of how you are going to react to it. You have a lot of information about your style at your fingertips already. This is empowering because you can act on it immediately. It doesn't require the participation of busy health care professionals or the health system. Frankly, you are already an expert at knowing yourself.

I have seen repeatedly that when people are facing an illness, especially when it comes to big issues, they tend to default to their natural style. Typically, their main personality traits and coping styles—good or bad—are consistent throughout their life, even if their illness worsens. In fact, as I mentioned earlier, most people's styles are amplified when facing a serious illness. Their personality traits and coping mechanisms become more pronounced as the stress or uncertainty in the illness increases. Knowing this can help you avoid unnecessary frustration.

Action 1: Assess Your Style

When I talk about styles, I am referring to a broad range of tendencies or personality traits when faced with different situations.

Everyone faces major life challenges in their own way. Certain dimensions are very relevant to navigating the illness journey. Below, I discuss these and highlight opposite ends of a spectrum in each. But humans are complex. People often find themselves somewhere in between, depending on the situation.

Information-seeking style: Some people are naturally curious and seek all the information they can. They read many books and enjoy figuring things out by themselves. They want lots of information in great detail. Others want very little information. They prefer to go to an expert, such as a doctor, to summarize it for them. They often like to be told the bottom line and ultimately what to do.

Receiving bad news: Some people don't like to talk about negative subjects and prefer to focus on the "positive." Others prefer to hear news straight up and face challenges head-on. They like direct information.

Planning into the future: Some people like to take things day by day. They often live in the moment and go with the flow. Others like to plan far into the future. They probably enjoy making detailed checklists and timelines for various activities. They want to control how things will unfold. They like things done in a certain way—their way or the highway. They plan things in detail so they can prepare for different scenarios.

Level of assertiveness: Some people are naturally reserved or shy, more introverted, and less likely to speak up, ask questions, or push back—especially if they prefer to avoid confrontation. Sometimes such people are labeled people-pleasers because they put others' needs before their own, whereas others are more extroverted and naturally talkative. They are open to speaking their minds, even if it makes others uncomfortable. They might be labeled assertive, direct, or blunt.

Coping mechanisms: When facing challenges, some people rely on healthy coping mechanisms such as meditation, yoga, going for walks, getting other exercise, or talking with friends. Other people have less healthy coping mechanisms, such as drinking, smoking, or stress eating.

Organization style: Not everyone is good at staying organized and keeping track of things. Some people tend to miss important dates or appointments. They may not be inclined to take notes to remember important details. Others may be much more organized, using notebooks, calendars, or organizer tools to keep track of appointments, medications, social obligations, and so on.

Need for privacy: Some people are private and may be very comfortable spending time alone. They don't share their emotions, and might even keep their diagnosis a secret from others. They may be more reluctant to ask for help and say no when people offer it. Others are more comfortable sharing news and emotions with many people. They enjoy spending time in large groups. They are fine with asking for and accepting help.

EXERCISE: REFLECT ON YOUR STYLE

The goal of this exercise is to uncover your individual style and natural tendencies when facing challenges. Reflect on your life and previous challenges you have faced—for example, the divorce of your parents, a relationship breakup, the loss of a loved one, a big exam. Or consider how you made an important decision, such as buying a house or car, having a child, or changing your career.

- Do you like to gather lots of information or do you prefer to learn as you go?
- Are you a long-term planner or a day-to-day kind of person?
- Do you deal with challenges head-on or do you prefer to wait for things to sort themselves out?
- What is your information-seeking style? When receiving serious information, do you like people to be direct or do you prefer to focus only on good news?
- What are your natural coping mechanisms? Think about your positive and negative tendencies.
- Do you like to consult with many people for advice or learn on your own?

The above are just examples of many possibilities. What is your natural style? What are your patterns?

Each Style Impacts the Journey Differently

We all have natural styles. Certain styles lend themselves better to maintaining control. And some styles put you more at risk of feeling out of control and more likely to end up in crisis. That said, every style has pros and cons. Every person will struggle in different ways.

For instance, people who like to live in the day-to-day, who are more passive when facing a challenge, and who find it difficult to advocate for themselves are at a high risk of not receiving the information they need to stay one step ahead of their illness. They will feel in the dark when changes are happening. They will often get swept up in the current of standardized care and feel overwhelmed because every change appears to be a major crisis.

In contrast, information seekers and super-planners who like to control situations and value their independence may feel frustrated in a health care system that doesn't encourage them to ask questions or provide open information. They risk forgetting to appreciate the joy in every day because they're so worried about planning for what-ifs in the future. They find it hardest when the illness affects their mobility and they can't do things for themselves because they are losing their autonomy, independence, and control.

I'm not suggesting you change your style, because no one style is the "right" style. Knowing your style, you can consciously identify potential pitfalls or likely challenges ahead and implement strategies to address any gaps. You can understand why you and people in your inner crew act the way they do and use this information to your advantage, even if it simply means understanding behaviors.

EXERCISE: UNDERSTAND YOUR NATURAL STRENGTHS

You can use the information about your natural patterns to your benefit. Consider the following:

- How will your style affect your illness experience? In what ways can you use your style to your benefit? What pitfalls or complications might arise because of your style?
- Also, look ahead and imagine: If your illness progresses, how will your style be amplified, and what will the consequences of that be?

Action 2: Assess Your Inner Crew's Style

Most people don't face an illness completely by themselves. The dynamics between a patient and their family members, or their inner crew, in the context of a serious illness makes the illness experience wildly unique. One of the reasons is that everyone has a different style.

Therefore, it is critical that you assess the styles of your inner crew—those who will be most involved in the care. How your inner crew's styles pair up or clash with yours is going to have a large influence on the journey.

I suggest you repeat the exercises in this chapter, imagining the answers for each of the key members of your inner crew. Consider how would they respond about themselves. Think about how they fared during challenges in their life. This will give you information about how they will behave on this illness journey with you. Ask them to complete the exercises for themselves, too.

Openly discuss and share your styles with one another in supportive ways. Let your crew know where you think you're going to need help, and listen to their thoughts about this. This is a powerful way to let people help in ways meaningful to you and to them. Being proactive in your journey this way may lend you a sense of more control.

Equally important is to share your style and your inner crew's styles with your health care team. Tell your doctors and nurses how you operate, especially your information-seeking style, and whether you like information straight up or not.

Conversation Starters: Here are some examples you can use to express your style to your health care team:

- "Doctor, I'm the kind of person who likes a lot of information. I like it straight up. Don't be afraid of breaking bad news. I may not like it at first, but with time, I will deal with it. More information gives me a sense of control. Information actually helps ground me."
- "Nurse, I prefer to defer to experts about what to do. I don't like confrontation or making decisions. Usually I leave it to my partner to make big decisions. In fact, we are a team, and you should be giving all important information to both of us so that we can discuss together. My partner is the quarterback of our team."

Action 3: Mix and Match

Whoever makes up your inner crew, they are the most obvious people to bolster potential weaknesses in your style. So that you have a better experience, ask yourself whom you need to do certain tasks. Mix and match the resources of your inner crew so that as one unit, you create a story that feels individual and reflects you and your family best.

For example, if you are a shy person, identify who in your inner crew will help you get all the information you need. Who is more of a go-getter? Who faces things head-on and asks a lot of questions? You need someone who isn't afraid to stand up for you and to advocate for things you believe in. If you are shy, you need someone you can rely on to gather information you need to prepare ahead.

If you tend to be disorganized, then ideally find someone in your inner crew who is rather the opposite—a good manager, organizer, and planner. This person can help you keep track of important information, appointment dates, medications, and so on.

Family Shout-Out: This process of mixing and matching doesn't have to be led by the patient. If you know that the patient has a hard time asking for help, instead of waiting for them to ask for it (which likely won't happen), you can offer specific assistance for something they need. Sometimes, for essential tasks like buying groceries or taking out the garbage, mixing and matching means completing those tasks for them.

Teng-Kee's Story: Knowing Your Style

My coauthor, Dr. Hsien Seow, has a personal story to illustrate this key in action. His uncle, Dr. Teng-Kee Tan, was diagnosed with inoperable pancreatic cancer and died a few years afterward. Teng-Kee was an extremely outspoken and gregarious person. When he got the diagnosis of pancreatic cancer, his wife, daughter (Sue), and son were not surprised that he quickly shared the news with all his friends and relatives. Sue said, "He would never be one to hide a serious illness. If anything, he overshares, which was his coping mechanism. He wanted everyone to know that he was sick—not to gain sympathy, but because that's how he is. He would be eating noodles in a Chinese restaurant and tell the waitress, 'I'm battling pancreatic cancer.' He was always that way. Whether he was ill or not, he liked to connect with other people. Part of that connection was telling people what he was going through." For him, it was easier to cope with the illness when he shared openly with those around him.

By leaning into his style, he exerted a sense of control over his illness story. For instance, because he wanted to be surrounded by love and support as he was dying, he actively invited his friends and family to visit as often as they could. Sue described it as his desire to have a "busy house—like in a perpetual kind of holiday mode." He spent time going through old photo albums so he could create a wall of favorite memories with all his closest friends and relatives—that way, he could literally be surrounded by people he loved. He even orchestrated a weekend when relatives from around the world flew in to have a living memorial celebration. He delivered his own eulogy, and the attendees celebrated stories from his life. It was Teng-Kee's way of exerting control over the dying process, finding peace and acceptance, and continuing to live on his own terms.

It is worth mentioning, though, that other members of his family have very different styles. His wife is an extremely private person. Sue explained that her mother is the type of person who would likely not tell others if she got sick. She'd feel that sharing a diagnosis would be burdening them with information. When a challenge arises, she wants privacy. She wants space to deal with it. But Sue and her brother handle things differently. On one hand, Sue is a more emotionally driven person. With her father, she focused less on the technical aspects of the disease and more on how to make her dad feel comfortable or her mom feel supported. She responds to crises through empathy. Sue's brother, on the other hand, is a solution-oriented person. He responds to crises by doing research. When he first learned of his father's diagnosis, Sue said, "he was immediately looking into the best place to get treated, the leading doctors, the latest clinical trials. He was forming a plan, calling his friends [who maybe knew] someone at this cancer center or that cancer center."

Sue felt that the family's different styles allowed them "to cover all the bases"—the technical and emotional. But there was also tension. "When you go through things like this, all your personalities get exaggerated because everybody's emotions are heightened. It's an extreme life situation. So all these things get dialed way up into overdrive." This was evident in how people coped. For instance, at times, the revolving door of visitors increased stress for Teng-Kee's immediate family, who were constantly hosting. Also, Teng-Kee was very open with Sue's young daughter about his disease. He would explain he was sick and receiving chemotherapy, and show her his chemotherapy pump. Some felt he might be oversharing and scaring his granddaughter. But even though she was a small child, he wanted her to know the truth of what was happening to him and to not be surprised when he wasn't there one day.

Sue said, "Some people reorient their life around the illness. My dad was not about that. His attitude was that this illness should orient itself around what he wanted to do." That was his style—control over how the experience played out. And the family embracing his style and understanding their own allowed them to make his last chapter meaningful. They collectively increased Teng-Kee's quality of life.

Know Your Style: Summary

- Your personality, how you face challenges, and how others in your inner crew have faced challenges in their lives will profoundly impact your illness experience, perhaps even more than the disease itself.
- Take time to reflect on and assess your own style and those of your inner crew members because everyone has strengths and weaknesses. Mix and match, as needed, with those in your inner crew who complement your style. Implement proactive strategies for outcomes you want.
- Share your style with your inner crew and health care team. Tell them how you want information, whom you have mixed and matched with, and whatever else you want them to know about your style.

5

CUSTOMIZE YOUR ORDER

“Knowing yourself is the beginning of all wisdom.”

ARISTOTLE

THE KEY Customize Your Order is about tailoring your care plan to match your goals and preferences. While the standard of care may be right for most people, at certain times you may want to modify your care to suit who you are as a unique individual.

Assumption: Doctor Knows Best

Most people assume that "doctor knows best." After all, doctors have gone to school for many years to become experts in specific illnesses and knowledgeable on all the cutting-edge research and treatment. At certain points during an illness, decisions will need to be made, like stopping or continuing with one treatment or trying another. Patients typically feel they should follow the doctor's recommendations. Often, they'll ask, "What would you do, doctor, in my situation?" or "What would you recommend if I were your relative?"

Unfortunately, too many people need care for the system to be able to truly offer individually tailored service. So doctors often default to offering the standard of care—a plan that has proved safe and effective—as the best choice. And patients end up following the recommended plan, or the standard of care, thinking it's the best for them. They go with the flow because, well, "doctor knows best."

Reality: You Are the Expert of You

The standard of care might be at odds with your preferences and values. As experts in their field, doctors will offer options based on the best standard care for your particular illness and based on your tests and scans. But they don't know you as well as you know yourself. They rarely have the time to unpack who you are in a deep way or to comb through the options with you to find the ones that best suit your preferences.

In other words, doctors may be good at offering personalized medicine, but they are not so good at offering personalized care. Personalized care is when the options are tailored to your individual needs, goals, and values.

Gary's Story: In the Dark

Gary was a patient with ALS. I had been caring for him for a few months, and his illness was causing a decline from month to month. Gary was very anxious about his breathing in general and extremely worried about what his breathing would be like as his condition worsened.

Later in his illness, Gary became suddenly breathless and was taken by ambulance to the hospital. He was admitted to the ICU, terrified, and agreed to be put on a breathing machine.

In the week following Gary's intubation, he wrote on his iPad that he wanted the breathing machine turned off. He felt he had made the wrong decision. It turns out that before the incident and his admission to the ICU, he and his wife had discussed the things he valued in life, among them his independence. He never wanted to be a burden to her. He told her he wouldn't want to use machines to breathe if his illness worsened to that point. However, when he became breathless suddenly, he did not know how to translate his values into a treatment decision. He ended up intubated on a breathing machine when this wasn't what he wanted.

Thankfully, Gary could still communicate his wishes in the ICU. Had he been in a coma or unable to communicate, his wife would have been faced with the heartbreaking decision of whether or not to keep him on machines, a profoundly difficult choice that no one ever wants to make for their loved one.

Consequences. If you don't know how to customize your order, you may begin to feel like just a number in the health care system rather than an individual, and that the care doesn't represent who you are. You become defined by the illness, not your unique qualities. Many patients have told me at the end of life that they felt their identity was lost, and that they no longer knew who they were. They felt they had lost their sense of autonomy and control. If you don't communicate your wishes, you are at high risk of receiving care you do not want.

Mo's Story: In the Know

I knew a patient, a young man with prostate cancer, named Mo. Mo recounted to me how difficult it was at the cancer center where he was receiving care: the oncologist kept trying to offer him different treatments that were excellent for prostate cancer but not in keeping with Mo's belief system. Mo had used only natural products throughout his life, and he wanted more natural-type treatments than the oncologist was offering. It became a huge source of tension between doctor and patient, and they were "butting heads all the time." Mo called it a "real tug-of-war."

Ultimately, Mo ended up getting another doctor because the first doctor just could not understand why someone so young did not want the chemotherapy that had been successful with so many other people. Mo still wanted to go to the cancer center to get support from the system, but he didn't want chemotherapy because he believed it was akin to putting poisons in his body. This was a core tenet of his belief system and he was adamant about staying true to his personal choices. While the doctor knew what the best standard treatment for the cancer was, Mo knew what was best for him.

Although this steadfastness fractured Mo's relationship with his doctor, it was more important for Mo to be true to himself. In choosing his own path, he made some trade-offs. He was aware that his choices might mean giving up a chance on the extended life that effective chemotherapy medicine might deliver. But even if the more natural methods did not work, Mo was prepared to accept that to stay true to his values.

Benefits. By remaining true to himself, Mo did not have to compromise his sense of self or his personhood. Mo knew himself so well that he knew what he was willing to trade off, which gave him a sense of control and autonomy. He was in charge of his choices, based on his values. He never had to face regret for receiving care that he did not want. This is the embodiment of person-centered care.

How to Customize Your Order

Customizing your order entails understanding how your personal preferences, wishes, and desires can be incorporated into your decision-making. A useful analogy is schools with uniforms. Every student at those schools must wear the uniform; this is non-negotiable. There are some options to choose from—pants, kilt, cardigan, sweater, vest—but by and large, the uniform choices are rather limited. However, every student wears their uniform a little bit differently. Some add their own personal flair. People tuck their hems and wear their kilt pins differently or their collars up or down, and so on. They find ways to make the uniform their own.

For life-changing illnesses, you are constrained by the health care system and the limits of medicine, but you can find ways to adapt the options to honor who you are. You might have to make trade-offs, but it's you who ultimately decides to make them.

I'm not suggesting that you direct all your care by demanding infinite tests, jumping the queue, or insisting on state-of-the-art procedures. There are limitations, just as with the school uniform. The doctor does know medical care best. But still, you can decide if what is being offered is what works best for you.

Here's an example: A cancer patient could be offered a chemotherapy treatment at the cancer center several times a week for four weeks in a row, and they might feel very nauseated the whole time. If the patient is at the beginning of the illness and the likelihood of drastically shrinking the tumor is high and maybe a cure is even possible, perhaps the patient would go for it. But if they are in a later stage of the illness, and this is the fifth line of chemotherapy (meaning they already tried four other chemotherapy regimens that eventually stopped working), and they realize time is limited, they might reconsider what they value most. If they value spending quality time with their family rather than commuting to and from the cancer center, they might choose not to take the chemotherapy.

Customizing your order is also about matching your overall treatment plans to what represents you as a person philosophically, spiritually, religiously, and culturally. Mo's example above shows his philosophical approach. He wanted to explore taking natural medicines. In some faiths, blood transfusions are against religious beliefs and this should be acknowledged as important to the patient. In some Indigenous cultures, smudging with sage and cedar baths are part of the healing cycle and ought to be incorporated into the care plan.

Not Just Treatment Decisions

People often think that preparing for future decisions is about specific treatment preferences, such as deciding about a feeding tube, a respirator, or cardiopulmonary resuscitation (CPR).

But customizing your order and infusing your values into decisions applies to more than medical decisions. It involves discussions about general values that are most important to you, such as trade-offs you are willing to make for the sake of more time. It is about prioritizing the few things you value most, whether that is your independence, the ability to communicate, spending time with family, quality of life, being social, or other priorities. Customizing your order is ultimately about ensuring you can achieve what you value. Your values should also inform the smaller moments that make up your day-to-day life. These in their totality define your quality of life.

Whether or not to go on a trip, quit your job, or move—these are decisions that affect your day-to-day life. Sometimes these life decisions may conflict with your values. For instance, a clinician might recommend a chemotherapy regimen that is every month for a year, which is grueling on the body. If you wanted to attend your son's graduation, you might skip a month (take a chemo holiday) to be strong enough to travel and attend the graduation.

Alternatively, sometimes there are ways to adapt how you will achieve what is important to you. I have seen people get weaker from their illness much faster than expected and fear they would not live long enough to be able to spend a holiday with family or attend an important wedding. So the families moved the wedding date up or celebrated the holiday early.

Many of the activities that are important to your overall happiness—such as social interactions, physical activity, work, and play—will likely be affected by your illness over time. Therefore, you need to consider how you will continue to maintain these activities, or modify them, to feel most like yourself throughout the illness.

Here are examples of customizing decisions:

- **Work/professional life:** You can decide whether to continue to work, take a leave of absence, or quit altogether.
- **Where to receive care:** You can decide to stay in your neighborhood or go outside of your city for care, and whether you want treatment in a hospital, at home, or in more than one place.
- **Investigations:** You can decide whether or not to continue more investigations, tests, or scans.
- **Treatments/drugs:** Some prescriptions or treatments may not be covered by your insurance and can be very expensive. Hardship due to the costs of treatment is sometimes referred to as financial toxicity. Customizing your order includes asking about whether there are affordable generic or alternative drug options.

If you're trying to personalize your care, don't be surprised if it's more challenging than you anticipated. Trying to tweak things can sometimes feel like working against the grain. And the bigger the decision, and the more incongruent your choice is to the standard of care, the bigger the bump you are likely to feel.

But I encourage you to keep trying to personalize your care. You will have to be a strong advocate for yourself if you want your care to reflect who you are. You are in charge of choosing your own path. And with every choice, there are trade-offs. The key is to be an informed consumer so you are making informed choices.

Invite your health care providers to talk to you about whether what they're offering fits into your own life. Share information about yourself: talk not just about physical issues but also about what's important to you and your life. For a smoother illness journey, consider doing this a little bit at a time throughout as opposed to waiting until late in the game, when many decisions have already been made.

Action 1: Think About Your Values and Goals

As mentioned, to customize your order, you need to reflect on your values; specifically, what is important to you and your quality of life. Knowing your values is like having a compass that guides you and your decision in the right direction.

For example, perhaps you greatly value extended time and living longer. This might mean trying all treatments, including experimental ones that could have impairing side effects and affect your ability to be independent. Or you might value quality of life more and be willing to trade off a potentially life-prolonging treatment for the ability to maintain independence and do the things you enjoy.

Tied into values are goals—goals are a way to live out your values. A goal is something you want to achieve, such as seeing a grandchild be born or attending a graduation or wedding. In some ways, the goal is the "what" and the value is the "why."

Once you define your values and goals, they can inform your decisions. For instance, you may feel strongly that you want to be cared for at home rather than in the hospital. The value behind that preference could be the desire to be around family in familiar surroundings. Or perhaps the value is to avoid high-technology interventions at end of life. Either way, the value will inform the decision about where to receive care, when the time comes to make that choice.

But this discussion about values and goals is not only about decision-making for precise medical situations. Eliciting your values is also about describing what gives meaning to your life and about what would make living no longer tolerable.

EXERCISE: DEFINE YOUR VALUES

In this exercise, you will start to define your values and goals, a personal set of guiding principles—a list of things that are most important to you and to defining who you are. Ask yourself:

- **What things do I value most?** Examples of values include spending time with family, the ability to communicate and keep mental faculties, maintaining independence and not being a burden on others, and maintaining privacy and dignity.

- **What are my biggest fears and worries about the future?** Examples of values expressed as fears include not being able to make independent decisions, having to ask others for help with basic needs like personal care (for example, bathing, dressing), and not being able to recognize or interact with people.

- **What activities are important to me that make life worth living and bring me joy?** For example: spending time in nature every day, doing my job, eating at new restaurants, and spending time with friends.
- **What am I most looking forward to doing in the future?** Examples of goals are attending a wedding or graduation, traveling to a favorite destination, and seeing the sunset or swimming in the ocean.

Write down your answers and refer to this list every time there is a decision, big or small.

Action 2: Apply Your Values to Your Illness Storyline

Customizing your order comes up in a very practical sense when you have to decide about treatments. Therefore, these reflections about your goals and values should be revisited over time. Your priorities, your preferences, and the trade-offs you are willing to make may change as the illness changes. So, to make sure you can customize your order, you must also zoom out with your medical team regularly so that your values and goals are considered in the context of where you are in your illness story.

People's values don't often change over time, but how they are applied to a person's life and decision-making might change based on which chapter of illness the person is in. For instance, if you are at a later stage in your illness, you may feel more tired and thus less willing to try treatments with high side effects to prolong your time. So, it's important also to check in with yourself and your inner crew throughout the illness, so that key values are factored into all decision-making.

Here are some points along the illness journey where you may want to check back in with your set of guiding principles:

- **Treatment decisions:** For example, when starting, continuing, or stopping a treatment; enrolling in a clinical trial; or having surgery.
- **Changes in the place of care:** For example, hospital, home, long-term care home, or hospice.
- **Changes in personal care:** For example, if you become unable to get to the toilet, get out of bed, shower, or go upstairs unassisted.
- **Financial decisions:** For example, whether it's time to quit a job, move, or sell a home.

Let's say that in your personal set of guiding principles, you determined that spending time with your family, maintaining your independence, and regularly playing cards with your friends are most important. Then every time you are faced with a decision such as trying a new treatment or enrolling in a clinical trial, you can check in against your personal set of guiding principles. You can ask yourself how the decision helps you achieve the things on your list. If the decision would risk too much on your list, or if you're not sure the trade-off will be worth it, you might decide not to proceed with it.

EXERCISE: ALIGN DECISIONS WITH YOUR VALUES

Especially when you are faced with a medical decision, remind yourself of your set of guiding principles. Ask yourself how your goals and values can inform your decisions. This self-reflection will help you make choices consistent with who you are and what you want to achieve. Here are questions to ask yourself:

- What is the decision to be made and what are the options?
- How do the different options align with my values?
- Which options will allow me to stay true to myself and what's important to me?
- Do the benefits outweigh the downsides/risks?
- What trade-offs am I willing to make?
- What am I unwilling to give up?
- Can any of the options be modified to match my values and goals? Can I negotiate this decision so it better matches who I am?

Action 3: Share Your Values

You will want to share and communicate your values to your inner crew so you are all on the same page. Sometimes there's tension between what a patient wants and what an inner crew wants. For instance, if you want to stop treatment because your body is tired, your family will be less likely to pressure you to continue treatment if they already know what's important to you. Expressing what you value now, in the big picture of your illness, is critical to helping your inner crew understand *the motivation* behind your decisions and preferences. It is the context that will help them better appreciate your intentions and better support your decisions, even if they would not make the same ones.

It's worth noting that your inner crew will also have their own unique values and goals—and those count, too. In some families, many decisions are made as a unit rather than by one person. With any decision, you may want to consider how it will affect the people in your life. Some decisions are a family affair because of the ripple effect on those around you. For example, say you want to be cared for at home no matter what because that's where you are most comfortable. If your needs are becoming such that the family has to care for you nearly 24/7 and are showing signs of serious burnout, this is where your values need to be considered, and frankly sometimes negotiated, alongside the inner crew's goals. So your preferences might cause tension when they conflict with the values or wishes of your family caregivers. Including them in decision-making and sharing your reasoning will help mitigate this.

Health Care Proxy or Substitute Decision Makers

Another reason that sharing your values with your inner crew is important is that there could come a time when you lack the mental capacity to make decisions on your own or are unable to speak for yourself.

If this happens, health care providers will look to the person who is designated to make decisions on your behalf. The term for this person or persons is different by region and country, but some of the more common terms are "health care proxy," "substitute decision maker," and "power of attorney for health care." It is important to learn what the relevant term is where you live and what the legal implications are of what they can and cannot do, as this differs by country, too.

Some of the most painful stories I hear are of family member health care proxies who must make decisions on behalf of a patient and don't know what the patient would have wanted. They often agonize over what they should or shouldn't do. They feel incredible guilt, doubt, or regret, which can last many years.

Therefore, your health care proxy is going to feel much more equipped to be in that role and make decisions on your behalf if you've shared what is important to you ahead of time. Talking about this early and often, which some people call "advance care planning," helps others understand what is important to you in various situations.

If for some reason you can't decide for yourself, you should understand who will be appointed automatically. And you will need to understand the process if you want the default person to be someone else. It is worthwhile investigating the laws where you live, as they can be nuanced and geographically specific.

Lastly, also make sure you express your values and goals to your health care provider team. This is important so that the providers can better make recommendations that fit your values. There may be options you're not aware of. This is how the illness journey can be more personalized.

EXERCISE: ASK THE PATIENT DIGNITY QUESTION

One way to express who you are to your health care providers is to ask yourself a modified version of the Patient Dignity Question developed by Dr. Harvey Max Chochinov, distinguished professor of psychiatry at the University of Manitoba. Ask yourself:

- What do providers need to know about me as a person to give me the best care possible?
- And then go to your next appointment and tell them: "Here's what you need to know about me to provide me the best care possible..." Alternatively, you can also tell them: "Here's what matters most to me..."

Wanda's Story: Customizing Your Order

To illustrate this key, I want to tell the story of Wanda, who cared for her daughter Cali. At six years old, Cali was diagnosed with diabetes and three separate heart conditions. Throughout Cali's illness, she and Wanda had to customize and personalize the standard of care to Cali's values, goals, and preferences.

From the beginning, Cali's conditions came with a long list of things she was told she could not do. The doctor said no to everything physical, including swimming, running, cartwheels, long walks, and dancing. The list went on and on.

Cali was clear about her values, even at six years old. "If I can't do that stuff, then what's the point?" she'd say to her mom. "Life is for living. These activities make me happy. These make my heart feel joy." Wanda was torn: she wanted to follow the doctor's orders but also understood Cali's point of view about how limited her life would be if she followed all the rules. Cali asked Wanda, "Is the point of life to follow these orders and just live in four walls?"

If they followed the doctor's rules, Cali wouldn't be able to walk to school (even though they lived a five-minute walk away). This was one of her favorite things to do with her friends—to walk to and from school and hang out along the way. She also loved dancing. There was a popular dance show on TV at the time and they were doing a special event in Cali's city. Cali was absolutely obsessed with the characters. Wanda emailed the organizers and asked if her daughter could come and watch because she couldn't participate. The organizers gave them a free ticket. When the day came, they invited Cali to participate on stage. Wanda's reaction was, "No way! This is high-level competitive dancing. You're not dancing." Cali looked Wanda and said, "Watch me." And she went right to the very front of the class. Wanda had brought a cardio defibrillator—they took it everywhere just in case—but she was still extremely nervous. She took photos and videos of Cali dancing on stage with everybody. And Cali told her parents many times, "That was the best day of my life."

In addition, Cali's parents' business meant they had to travel occasionally. Even though the doctors told them they always had to be within one hour of the pediatric hospital in case something happened with Cali, her parents made the personal decision to take their daughter with them on work trips. They traveled to many places. Wanda confided, "Looking back, our best memories were of traveling to places that she would never have experienced if we had listened to the doctors." There are always risks to be weighed and trade-offs to be made, but Cali and her parents applied their preferences to the recommendations.

Moreover, sometimes customizing your order isn't easy, especially when there is pushback from the health care system to follow the status quo. When Cali turned eleven, the family was told—in a way that felt totally out of left field—that she needed a heart transplant. The doctor handed them a booklet titled "When Your Child Needs a Heart Transplant." They were dumbfounded. Wanda recalled, "It was definitely quiet in the elevator back down to the parking garage. And about halfway home, Cali finally piped up and said, 'I don't want a heart transplant.' And that was the first time she really said that."

The push from the pediatric hospital to do a heart transplant was strong. Their doctor was forceful and insistent. She was the head of the transplant team and would often cite her research and statistics about the benefits of the transplant. As Cali's illness worsened, the family had to seriously revisit her values and wishes and weigh the pros and cons of the transplant.

They read the booklet and did research online. Cali learned many facts about having a transplant and pointed out that her three combined heart conditions made her specific transplant far more complicated. It may have been the best medical option, but Wanda recalls the tension around it, because Cali was not convinced. Cali told her mother that she didn't want another person to die for her to live. Even though Wanda explained this was a heart from someone who had already passed away, Cali felt adamant that this was not a route she wanted. Of course, her parents wanted Cali to understand the severity of the situation and they continued to have more discussions.

Cali ultimately agreed to begin initial tests for a transplant. Unfortunately, she passed away suddenly before she could have the surgery. Wanda said, "No matter what your condition—a heart condition, cancer, or any other illness—it's your right to do what's best for you. Ultimately, you know yourself best. And doctors should listen."

Customize Your Order: Summary

- You can tailor your care plan to your personal values and goals; therefore, determining what those are is important. When you receive new information or when decisions need to be made, consider how the available choices match up with your values and goals.
- Communicate your values and goals to your inner crew and health care providers so they can support you in making decisions that are aligned with what you want.
- Your goals and preferences might change as you arrive at forks in the road along your illness journey. Revisit the questions about what's important to you at each juncture. This way, you'll maintain control of your experience and move from having a generic experience to one that's more personalized.

6

ANTICIPATE RIPPLE EFFECTS

“For every action, there is an equal and opposite reaction.”

SIR ISAAC NEWTON

THE KEY Anticipate Ripple Effects is about appreciating the parallel journey of those around you. Imagine tossing a small stone in a still lake. From where the stone drops, the water ripples out in widening concentric circles. In the same way, your family members, friends, neighbors, colleagues, and others in your life experience the ripple effect of your illness.

Assumption: It's All about You

Most people assume that it's all about you, the patient; that you should receive all the energy and attention from your health care providers. To the health system, you are the main star of the illness experience. Your inner crew, your chosen family, will do nearly anything for you because they love you and you are sick. They will rally around you. I hear people say things like, "I would have done anything for my sick spouse" or "It was their wish, so I had to fulfill it."

Reality: Others Are on a Parallel Journey with You

It is very unusual for a patient to go through an illness alone. Usually, an inner crew of family and friends supports them. The inner crew often experiences both the person's illness journey and their own, often with some physical and emotional toll.

This parallel journey is unique and occurs in the shadows of a patient's experience. The inner crew's needs are often overlooked. Family members often feel guilty drawing attention to their own needs, since they feel that the patient's needs should be the priority. After caring for a patient for a long time, family members have told me, "I lost my sense of me."

Michelle's Story: In the Dark

Michelle was twenty-three years old, ambitiously pursuing continued studies and working full time. Then she learned her mother was diagnosed with a metastatic cancer, originating in the breast but now spread to the brain and lung. "For two years," Michelle said, "my life was on hold."

For a period, she was commuting long distance because she could manage the medications and care for her mother around working hours. But in the final period, she was given permission to work from home. She spent her days changing her mother's diapers, giving baths, taking her to appointments, and giving medication. Plus, she worked more than eight hours a day from home. This lasted for many months.

Michelle had not anticipated the ripple effect, and it took its toll. She told me, "I wish I'd understood what I was supposed to do for me and what I was supposed to do for her... The hardest part is when you have been consumed by the needs of the other and cannot see yourself anywhere any longer. I didn't have the capacity to be me. You live giving all you are for another person."

Consequences. Because Michelle was not fully prepared for the role she undertook in helping her mother, she experienced a loss of her own personhood. In her own words, she was losing herself in the role of caregiver. She constantly felt unprepared and in crisis-prevention mode. She wasn't able to make space for this major commitment. It felt reactive rather than proactive. While she loved her mother dearly, she wished the experience felt more like a gift than an obligation, one she was willingly and knowledgeably signing up for.

Kenisha's Story: In the Know

When Mira was diagnosed with advanced cancer, Kenisha, her wife of many years, was devastated. But friends and family came in droves to offer Kenisha a hand. Instead of declining offers, Kenisha always said yes. This wasn't easy for her, as she was a private and independent person. However, Kenisha knew that the only way she would survive was to continue to stay busy with work while coordinating a well-orchestrated support team for Mira.

Over a period of weeks after Mira's diagnosis, Kenisha had taken up neighbors, friends, and family on their kindnesses. She had friendly visitors to accompany Mira outside for walks or to have coffee. She had dog walkers and dog sitters for their beloved pet. She always had meals in the fridge and freezer. She had drivers and delivery people. She activated her village and created a community of support around Mira. This allowed her to take care of herself as well.

Kenisha created an inner care circle and an extended care circle. In the inner crew were Mira's siblings and family as well as a few close friends. The next layer contained more family, neighbors, colleagues, and friends. Once activated, her village made the journey better for her and for Mira.

Kenisha tried her best to keep her life as normal as possible while staying true to herself. She did not forgo her own appointments and social opportunities. To stay at home 24/7 trying to do it all would have frustrated Mira and worn out Kenisha. When she was with Mira, Kenisha could enjoy creating memories—and be in the role of wife, not always a task-driven caregiver.

Benefits. Because Kenisha anticipated that she was going to experience ripples from the start, she prepared early and avoided finding herself exhausted at the end of the journey from juggling all the tasks and trying to be the person who did everything. She knew to ask for help and involve others (who also experienced the ripples) in ways they could be helpful. She activated a community of care that wrapped around her and Mira. She continued working. In fact, she found it invigorating to be at work. Kenisha felt she was keeping her head above water, even though she was working full time and caregiving. She was better able to enjoy her time when she was with Mira, giving her happiness rather than feeling burned out.

How to Anticipate Ripple Effects

Those who have a relationship with you will be affected in some way—some more profoundly than others. Like ripples in water, those closest to you, your inner crew (in the center, or first ring; see figure 5), will be the most impacted. Others will fall in different degrees of impact (the second and third rings) depending on their involvement in your journey. The concentric rings in figure 5 are a way to represent how emotionally close and connected people are to you and the extent of the ripple effect of your illness on them. Even those who are close to you but are not involved in helping manage the illness—for instance, young children—will be affected.

The Ripple Effect

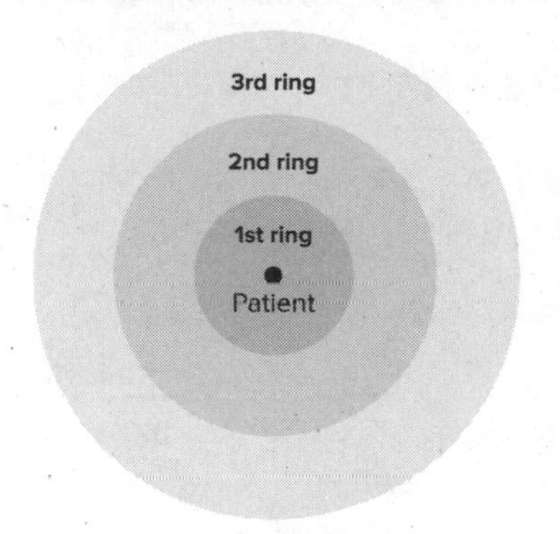

FIGURE 5.
Those closest to the patient in the center will be impacted the most

You'll want to consider how your illness will affect these people in your life across the various rings of the ripple effect. Appreciate that everyone's reactions and styles are different. Some might require additional supports (for example, children may want to talk to counselors about having a sick parent).

Once you acknowledge that there are people who will be affected by your illness, you can consider that there are people in those rings, most likely from the inner crew, who will have instrumental roles in your illness journey, ranging from emotional and social support to physical and personal care. Some will lean into those roles and some will lean out. Leaning in means they will actively help you in different ways. If people lean out, it does not necessarily mean that they do not care for you. Life-changing illnesses affect people in different ways. People cope in different ways. People have competing priorities. A person's style will also influence whether they lean in or lean out.

As the patient, it's worth appreciating that your illness may change over time, and that also means your needs may change over time. So people can lean in and out over time, or take on different roles, depending on your situation.

EXERCISE: MAP THE RIPPLE EFFECT

It is helpful to map out the ripple effect of your illness by explicitly naming who will be affected and to what degree.

First ring: Typically includes spouse, children, best friends—your chosen family (those most close and connected to you, physically and emotionally). Note that the number of people in a person's inner crew will naturally differ. You want to identify those who naturally are the closest layer of people in your life already, who may or may not be blood-related.

Names of people in the first ring (inner crew/first ripple):

____

____

Second ring: Typically includes extended family and friends (those you are also close with but who are not your "chosen family").

Names of people in the second ring (second ripple):

____

____

Third ring: Typically includes neighbors, coworkers, and social and community networks (i.e., those you might socialize with occasionally).

Names of people in the third ring (third ripple):

___

___

The Label of Caregiver or Carer

Much of what those who lean in are doing is called caregiving. Even though they may think of their role as spouse, child, sibling, or best friend, they now also have the role of family caregiver (also called family carer). Sometimes they are called informal caregivers to differentiate them from formally trained and paid caregivers. Knowing the caregiver label and using it to search for information, you can identify resources and supports that can be helpful early in the illness.

While many people may not identify as a caregiver or understand the term, they are, in fact, everywhere in society. More than one in four Canadians are currently caregivers (eight million individuals), and nearly half will become one in their lifetime. US statistics are similar. A 2020 national US survey conducted by the AARP and the National Alliance for Caregiving (NAC), estimated that one in five Americans (fifty-three million individuals) is providing unpaid care to an adult with health or functional needs, each spending an average of twenty-four hours per week providing care.

The Burdens and Joys of Caregiving

Caregivers and the role of caregiving is complex. Many people willingly step into and stay in the role. Some do it because they feel a sense of love or responsibility. They tell me, "I wouldn't have it any other way." But there are times when they support the patient's needs because of guilt, obligation, and duty. It is not always done happily or by a loved one.

I think it is fair to say that the caregiver role can be both a responsibility and a joy at the same time. It feels like a responsibility, sometimes even a burden, because most of the support you will require is going to fall outside the walls of the hospital. Research shows that approximately 75 to 80 percent of people's care occurs outside a hospital and is performed by the informal caregivers in a patient's home. That said, many caregivers describe the experience as a gift. One caregiver told me: "It has been the hardest thing I've done in my life, but the most rewarding." They wouldn't trade the experience for anything because it made the relationship closer. It is a special time that they otherwise wouldn't have had. They use the time to make memories, find closure, and demonstrate what loving and caring look like to each other.

Every situation and patient-caregiver dynamic will be different. What I have experienced is that caregivers are happier and more grounded when they know what they're getting into and can stay ahead of the game. When they are in the know, plan ahead, and draw on other people to help, they are less overwhelmed and more able and willing to provide support to the patient. They are able to experience more of the joys of caregiving and fewer of the burdens.

Tip: The more your caregiver leans into your diagnosis, the more your illness will affect their life. For many patients I meet, this causes them to feel like a burden. Other patients do not consider their inner crew's needs at all. But it is important to recognize that your inner crew often may not feel they have permission to speak up for themselves and ask for what they need. They will likely experience a great deal of emotion along their parallel journey, including while trying to care for themselves. Therefore, make space for your caregivers to process. At medical appointments, allow them space to ask questions. Check in to make sure they have the time they need. Encourage them to take care of their own needs and practice self-care.

Family Shout-Out: Caregivers have a critical role in the health of the patient. And they have their own health care needs, too. As a caregiver, you will fare better if you are positioned front and center, as well. You deserve the same opportunity as the patient to prepare for this life-changing role. Knowing ahead of time what the caregiver position will entail—physically, emotionally, financially, spiritually—will better prepare you to stay ahead of the game. Now is the time to look for relevant resources, such as support groups, local or national caregiver organizations, books, and so on. Resources enable you to be in the know and increase the likelihood that you will feel more of the joys and fewer of the burdens of caregiving.

Action 1: Identify Your Primary Caregiver

Typically, within your inner crew, one person will consistently lean in and be there for you throughout the entire illness. This is your go-to person for your care (for example, your spouse). This person, your primary caregiver, has your back. Or you might have a few primary caregivers—for example, if the duties are shared among a few adult children or close friends. They will be the eyes and ears for you when you aren't being monitored by the formal health system.

It is important to ensure that your primary caregiver knows what they're signing up for. If they feel unexpectedly "volunteered" for the primary caregiver role rather than having been able to consciously sign up for it, they will be at higher risk of burnout.

Anticipating ripple effects is about appreciating that while you are the star of your illness, your primary caregiver is a supporting character who plays a vital role. As the patient, your role is to help them understand what to expect and to prepare them. It is like rehearsing before the actual event, so that you and your primary caregiver can develop a proper plan early on. This will make it easier for them to manage their responsibilities.

Tip: In many ways, you and your primary caregiver should be considered a unit. Your caregivers and inner crew must be recognized as having a critical role in supporting you. Inform your health care providers of your primary caregiver and what role you want them to play. This includes explicitly explaining which health information they can or cannot be told.

EXERCISE: IDENTIFY YOUR PRIMARY CAREGIVER

Relook at the names of the people you listed as affected by your illness (page 122). Identify who among those in your inner crew you would consider to be your primary caregiver. Make time to have an explicit discussion with that person about what you need from them and what they might need to do this role.

Action 2: Review the Job Description

Too often, being a caregiver is like taking a job without knowing the job description. Many family caregivers have no formal training in health care, nor have they ever received instructions or guidance, so when they take on the role, they don't truly understand the many ways in which caregiving is going to affect their life.

Here, I try to provide a very generic job description. Note that the roles and responsibilities depend on your illness and specific needs as a patient, which can change over time. But below are some of the major categories of tasks that caregivers take on—often not realizing that these count as caregiving:

- **Psychological, emotional, and social support:** For example, providing moral or peer support; checking in by phone; making social, in-person visits; taking you to leisure activities; and providing a break for other caregivers.
- **Transportation, information seeking, and coordination of appointments:** For example, accompanying you to appointments, arranging medical appointments, keeping track of medical information, and finding out about available services.

- **Financial/legal affairs:** For example, banking and paying bills, doing taxes, and arranging legal documents such as wills or power of attorney.
- **Help around the house:** For example, getting prescriptions, grocery shopping, cooking, cleaning, laundry, yard work, and so on. These are referred to as instrumental activities of daily living.
- **Personal care:** For example, dressing, lifting, feeding, bathing, toileting, and hygiene. These are referred to as activities of daily living.

This list of tasks is reinforced by the AARP-NAC survey referenced earlier. Their survey of current caregivers found that all helped with tasks such as transportation, grocery shopping, housework, preparing meals, and managing finances and medications. Most caregivers helped with a few personal care tasks such as feeding, bathing, toileting, getting dressed, and assisting in moving in and out of beds or chairs. More and more were assisting with medical or nursing tasks, advocating for services, and coordinating between and communicating with health care professionals.

However, this snapshot survey gives the impression that caregiving is a full-out sprint from the start. What I have found, though, is that caregiving responsibilities grow slowly over time. Particularly for those who are caregiving over long periods, the needs typically change so slowly that any increasing demand is sometimes hard to notice.

This is what a typical story might look like: From the start, families naturally become informal cheerleaders. They rally around the patient and provide emotional and moral support. They take on a few tasks to help here and there. As the illness changes, they start driving the patient to appointments and doing errands. Then they get involved in grocery shopping, banking, and cleaning. Eventually, caregivers are needed more, shifting from errands to providing more personal care. This may include toileting, bathing, feeding, and dressing.

Here especially, when helping with activities of daily living, caregivers often scramble to balance the needs of the patient and their own family/personal needs. Many caregivers are also working full time and/or caring for others (parents, spouses, or children) simultaneously. Many stop exercising, socializing, working, and participating in hobbies to care for their loved one. With no end in sight, caregivers easily burn out, having given up the things that sustained them. They are at higher risk of anxiety, depression, and even mortality. And what I often see is that when the family members struggle, the patient's suffering is amplified. Sometimes the caregivers themselves become unwell—quietly, in the shadows of the patient's illness. And then you could have multiple ill people in one illness experience.

As the patient, you should appreciate that depending on the illness and your needs, being a caregiver can feel like running a marathon. Deciding to run a marathon requires you to train, have a sense of how long the race will take, and have a support system around you. You prepare yourself mentally and physically to do this. Unlike a sprint, it is often a very long journey and you need to pace yourself. In the US, the AARP-NAC national survey data shows that the average duration of caregiving is four and a half years, and three out of ten caregivers have provided care for five years or longer.

So again, ideally, discussions about who your primary caregiver is should be done early and intentionally. They should understand what roles you are asking them to play and how their individual skills in life can be used to support you.

Expectations should be revisited and renegotiated periodically. And it's fair for a caregiver to ask for help or to lean in and out depending on what is being asked of them.

Family Shout-Out: Being a primary caregiver will impact your life. There can be profound joys that come from caregiving. But it can also feel like a burden and responsibility. Space must be made for the caregiver role, especially if you are already quite busy. Make your choice to be a caregiver an informed decision. Ideally, do all the exercises in this book along with the patient. Consider how taking on the role will affect your relationship with the patient; your relationship with your partner/children/family; your health; your career/job; your social life; your finances; and your future. And ask yourself these questions when considering taking on the role:

- Do I understand the big picture of the patient's condition? Do I understand the full scope of the changing caregiving role from diagnosis to end of life?
- What does the patient want and need?
- How much and what type of care do I want to provide? What are my skills and resources?
- What am I able and comfortable to do, and uncomfortable or unwilling to do?

Action 3: Activate Your Village

Just like the saying "it takes a village to raise a child," it takes a village to care for someone who's sick. Activating your village involves tapping into the informal system of care, support, and guidance that already surrounds you and your family. It is about consciously harnessing the connections that exist in your family, social, and community spheres. It involves asking for help or accepting offers from people in your various networks of support. It can also include hiring help, if that's an option.

This is important because many caregivers try to do it all themselves and say no to help from others, which leaves them at high risk of burnout. As a patient, you have a responsibility to know the common tasks of being a caregiver, which are outlined in the previous section, and to know when more help may be necessary.

Proactively discuss, negotiate, and generate your village with your main caregiver. Together, consciously look at all the various tasks you need or will need help with. And mark out what roles your caregiver is doing and what roles you could get support for. Depending on the nature of your condition, your needs will likely change over time. As such, periodically revisit whom you have activated in your village, because these roles may need to be renegotiated.

EXERCISE: ORGANIZE YOUR VILLAGE

Review the names you listed in the "Map the Ripple Effect" exercise (page 122) and the tasks in the "Review the Job Description" section (page 127). Identify who could help with which tasks, recognizing that your primary caregiver alone cannot do all tasks. Below is an example of what your task list could look like. However, personalize it to your needs and situation.

Task	Name
Grocery shopping	Maya (sibling)
Pick up prescriptions	Micah (child)
Accompany to doctor visits	Jordan (spouse)

After you've created this task list, engage each person on the list in formal conversations to ensure they are willing and able to help with the desired tasks. This also helps them see who else is in the network of support.

Family Shout-Out: You might feel a wide range of emotions such as anger, sadness, and guilt throughout the illness. Know that this is common, and it is good to acknowledge these feelings. People often find that talking with other caregivers who face similar conditions is beneficial. Your goal as a caregiver is to try to make sure the patient is safe, clean, and comfortable. If they are, rest assured that you have done your job. Strive for balance, not perfection.

To sustain your role as a caregiver and avoid burnout, take care of yourself first, just like Kenisha did in the story earlier in this chapter. Try to be intentional and proactive about self-care and finding strategies to stay resilient. Here are three ways you can support your own resilience:

- **Educate yourself about the role:** The more you understand the patient's condition, are in the know, have zoomed out, and know your styles, the more prepared you will be for whatever happens.
- **Plan ahead:** Planning for contingencies and letting others in the inner crew know what their roles will be can help mitigate the impact of unexpected and chaotic surprises. Having a schedule (even if you aren't the one making the schedule) and tools to keep people organized will ensure everything runs smoothly. Delegating and clearly communicating the plans will help you avoid misunderstandings.
- **Prioritize your own health:** To the best of your ability, focus on eating well, resting, doing physical activity, and taking breaks.

A final note about your self-care as a caregiver: Patients often feel they are a burden to their inner crew, especially their primary caregivers. If you run yourself ragged, you might actually contribute to the patient's sense of burden. So this is a reminder that not only does practicing self-care and meeting your needs reduce your risk of burnout and negative health issues, but it can also greatly assuage the patient's sense of guilt.

Signs of Burnout

Both patient and caregiver have a role in preventing caregiver burnout. There are lots of existing resources, such as peer support groups, blogs, and community organizations that either can be a support group or provide information and advice about caregiving. Look for these early on.

Also, as a patient, it is useful to remember that many times caregivers don't get a big break from caregiving. Rarely do caregivers aim to take a long vacation from caregiving, but they do want and need to take little sips of self-care along the journey. Try to consciously allow them to take small breaks to sustain themselves and stay resilient. A small break could be a moment for relaxation, a walk outside, a coffee with a friend. It will look different for every person. Collectively, these moments can be an effective way for caregivers to stay grounded. Check in with your caregiver. You are a team.

Here are signs of burnout you and your caregiver can look out for:

- Irritability
- Insomnia
- Loss of appetite
- Crying
- Fatigue
- Lacking compassion
- Losing weight
- Feeling constantly stressed
- Not doing things they enjoy
- Doing most of the caregiving tasks alone
- Not asking for or accepting help from others

If your caregiver exhibits these signs, seek out resources, programs, and services to support them. As a patient, you should encourage your caregiver to also see their health care provider about their own experience and address their own health needs. As well, the caregiver should revisit all the keys in this book and apply them to their role.

Isabelle's Story: Anticipating Ripple Effects

To illustrate this key, let me introduce Isabelle, who was a caregiver for her older sister, Julie. When Julie was first diagnosed with breast cancer, she was thirty years old and a single mother of a toddler. Isabelle ended up caring for her sister for seven years, including at the end of life.

When I asked Isabelle if the metaphor of the ripple effects resonated with her, she said, "You don't choose to become a caregiver, it just happens." She talked about how caregivers are "an extension of the patient... They trust us when everything is out of control." When you're a caregiver, it is easy to neglect yourself. She recalled, "When somebody is ill and in bed and not able to get up, you can't put it on pause." Being a caregiver affected all aspects of Isabelle's life, such as deciding to work part time and then quitting work altogether as Julie's needs changed.

We also spoke about the various roles she had to take on. She told me: "The health care system does not prepare you to be a caregiver." She added, "The doctors hardly even looked at me, even when I was next to her." So Isabelle had to learn to advocate for her sister, and to "walk through the hospital doors and be ready to ask for what [was needed] and to climb a mountain" if that was required. Her roles included being the day and night nurse, managing fluids and oxygen; acting as a pharmacist dealing with pain and anxiety medications; being the transport service for appointments; being the cook; being the social worker to support the entire family's waves of emotion; and being an aunt to her niece. She was the overall "crisis manager" for her sister, an all-consuming role that never had days off.

Isabelle knew how critical her mental health was and paid attention to signs that she needed help: "[I looked for] little red flags—when I was completely forgetting about myself, when I would need a little break, or when we needed to bring somebody else in the circle." What I call "the village," she called "the spider web" of different people to help with different aspects of daily life. Communicating with the spider web was critical. This group of family and friends made meals, did school drop-offs, drove Julie around, and ran other errands. "You need to know whom to talk to, when; who can come, who cannot," Isabelle told me. When you need help over a long period, there are ups and downs and needs vary. Isabelle said, "Even as willing and good-hearted as people can be, they're not living in the house."

When I asked what she thought about self-care, Isabelle said, "It's a very hard question. Because there are different stages. When she was stable, I could be attentive to myself. But when we were in crisis and she wasn't able to be herself, I had to advocate for her. It wasn't the time to think about myself. I have to admit, I completely lost myself. I want to let other people know that that can happen. You don't realize how tired you are mentally. Everybody has their own method of how to cope. You have to try to find a balance."

Near the end of her sister's life, there were many times Isabelle felt utterly unprepared for what to expect next. At one point, a home care nurse asked Isabelle if she could still care for Julie at home. She answered, "Yes, for today! But tomorrow, I don't know." Even though home care nurses provided Julie with some care, their main role was to teach Isabelle how to do most of the care on her own. She confided, "In the moment of crisis, you have no limits. Reflecting on it all, I wish I was told where the limit was." In the last week of Julie's life, her doctor said to Isabelle, "You can just be her sister now." Isabelle broke down at those words because she realized that up to that point, she'd had to do so much that she'd had no time to simply be Julie's sister.

Ultimately, Isabelle shared her story to remind us of what she learned from her experience: "People are scared to talk about end of life. And even when you're in the hospital, the doctors, nurses, or social workers don't talk about it. They whisper about it. Nobody has a good discussion about it. So patients and families are not prepared." We have to change that and not be afraid to plan for the future, including dying, so we can embrace life while we are still living.

Anticipate Ripple Effects: Summary

- Your life-changing diagnosis will impact those around you in a ripple effect, with those closest to you being impacted the most.
- Usually a few key people in the inner crew take on a large role in the patient journey. They are called caregivers and what they do is called caregiving.
- Caregivers need to know the job description of caregiver and where they need more training or help from others. They need support to take care of themselves, too.

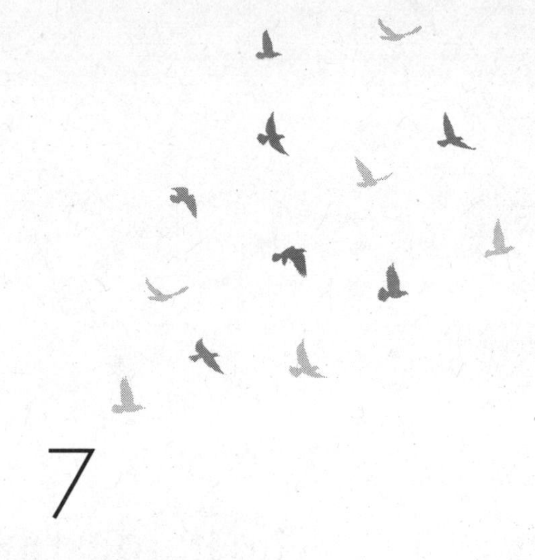

7

CONNECT THE DOTS

“The hardest part about directing is getting everyone on the same page.”

ROBERT MARSHALL

THE KEY Connect the Dots is recognizing that you and your inner crew need to make the links between fragmented health care providers. You also need to be messengers bringing vital information from your private world to the health care system to retain your sense of self and control throughout the journey.

Assumption: The System Will Lead Coordination

Most patients assume that navigation and coordination are embedded into the roles of their health care providers. They think that it's a relatively well-connected system and that the right hand knows what the left is doing. In this modern era, patients assume that each health care team has access to what the other team is doing—perhaps with an electronic patient chart that shares everything among the teams. They think their information arrives ahead of them regardless of where they next land, and that their health care providers pass the information along smoothly, like quarterbacks of the illness journey. They assume they can just pick up where they left off with a previous doctor without having to repeat information. And they think their various doctors and health care teams have the regular opportunity to read their files beforehand and huddle to plan for the care.

Reality: Someone Must Manage Your Illness Journey

The reality is that the health care system is complex and complicated, spread across a series of organizations and independent providers. There are a lot of moving parts behind the scenes.

Every health system has an ever-expanding variety of strategies to coordinate to make your care smoother and more seamless. These may include patient navigators, care coordinators, electronic medical records, text alerts, email reminders, and so on. All of these are meant to connect parts of the system that can then be connected to you and your family.

However, despite best efforts, there is no perfect system. Things can fall through the cracks. That is why it is not uncommon, at some point, for a care provider to ask what happened at the last visit, and for the patient to be surprised and thinking, "Don't they talk to each other?"

Perhaps the lack of connection isn't as obvious within just one specialist team. A single specialty team is responsible for one aspect of your care. They are specialists in an organ system or a particular illness. For example, the cardiology team is responsible for the issues related to the heart; the nephrologist is responsible for the kidneys.

However, it is typical for people to be cared for by multiple specialist teams and to experience different care settings (for example, office, clinic, hospital, home, nursing home, or hospice). This is when the communication, collaboration, and coordination between the teams is highly variable; often, the specialist teams do not have any opportunity to speak to other teams, or information arrives too late. It can feel as if they work independently of one another.

Beyond the information-sharing aspects of the health system, from a human side of things, care can also feel fragmented. Because of the complexity of all the moving parts, it is easy to lose your sense of self. Someone (and this someone could be you, depending on your style) needs to take on a managerial role, not just to coordinate information but also to ensure that the key parts of your story are not lost in the information shuffle. Like all patients, you need someone to be the glue to hold the different parts of the system together and to weave your personal details into the care. This will allow you to retain your sense of self and to feel more in control.

Michael's Story: In the Dark

I once interviewed a man named Michael, who cared for his mother, Phyllis. She was diagnosed with kidney cancer, which was treated with radiation. But she had a lot of pain. As a result, she was in and out of the emergency department, which led to several hospital admissions.

Michael said it felt as if he were always driving the bus, telling the medical professionals what the issues were since no one was addressing the root cause of the pain. The hospital usually wanted to discharge her quickly and free up the bed. After one hospitalization, Phyllis was sent home with ten hours of home care support a week, which was insufficient to allow her to live independently at home. Phyllis lived alone. Michael and his sister worked full time. He wondered, "What am I going to do on the weekends? What am I going to do at night?" He quickly realized his new role. "All of a sudden, I was the caregiver," he said. "I was in charge of somebody who's got all these conditions. She didn't come home with the flu. She had cancer."

Organizing her care was a nightmare. He felt like the "chief, cook, and bottle washer," doing all the tasks. He said, "You're on the phone, you're chasing people—you're trying to get nurses back, you're trying to get the doctor back. I'm on the phone with the pharmacist. She had twelve prescriptions. Plus, you get these people that are overworked, understaffed; some are not trained properly." This game of what Michael called "monkey in the middle" continued with the family doctor, the on-call doctor, and the nurses, until Phyllis eventually passed away a few weeks later. Her pain was never managed. Ultimately, Michael was so frustrated because he expected that the system would be coordinated, but his experience was the opposite.

Consequences. There are multiple consequences of assuming that things are coordinated when they're not. Patients and families feel like the care is chaotic. All the juggling causes people to feel frustrated and overwhelmed. Important information is missing or lost. Medical mistakes can occur. Wrong or unwanted care is delivered. Everything feels reactive.

Mary Anne's Story: In the Know

Mary Anne was a mother and caregiver to her only son, Tyler, who had a mental illness. Right from the start, Mary Anne had to connect the dots of the health system to get a correct diagnosis. Initially, they thought Tyler's lack of motivation and signs of depression were a result of recreational marijuana use and typical teenage angst. The family doctor prescribed antidepressants. Tyler saw a social worker and was taking the medications, but he was not getting better. He eventually dropped out of high school and got a job in a fast-food chain.

Mary Anne told me she's the type of person who will ask questions and will expect answers. But even then, she consulted a lot of different people in the community and in the health care system but "wasn't getting any answers." After several years, Tyler confided in her that he had suicidal thoughts, and she took him to the emergency department. Mary Anne pushed for Tyler to have a psychiatrist assess him, and he was given the proper diagnosis of schizophrenia. This enabled Tyler to enter a long-term hospital-based rehabilitation program. He worked hard for nearly a year and was released from the program.

Mary Anne knew she had to be much more involved with his health care and mental health care. She needed to take charge because she realized there were "no community services to support him." She told me, "I needed to bust my way in to get information so I could help him." She had to get not only information about the illness, but also information about health care, about resources or lack of resources, about how to deal with his health care provider, and about how to deal with his financial situation. She said, "It's multidimensional and it's complex and it goes on for a lifetime."

Even when he was in the treatment programs, Mary Anne called Tyler regularly to check in on him, sometimes every day. If there were issues, she problem-solved with Tyler, and called his nurses, the program staff, and the director to find workable solutions and provide appropriate care. She acted as the glue to make sure everyone knew their roles, including Tyler and herself, in his care plan. Mary Anne admitted, "I was the manager, you know." She would manage any issues that Tyler faced.

Benefits. Knowing early on that you need someone to play a coordinating role in your care will increase the likelihood that things won't fall through the cracks, that you will receive the care you need, and that your care experience will be more organized. It helps ensure you will get access to resources when you need them, and that someone is advocating for your best interests. It allows you to get not only the best but also the most personalized care since it is how you can tailor the care plan to your situation.

How to Connect the Dots

Connecting the dots is realizing that even though the health care system has many strategies to coordinate information, there are still elements of care that are siloed. Not all your information will be passed along in the medical charts, even if it's an electronic medical record, because very often pieces of information in your chart are held by different parts of the health care system. Sometimes different providers and settings do not have access to the same electronic systems or use the same software and cannot access the record. Human error occurs, too.

This means that you and your family have a role in coordinating information across different clinicians and care teams, such as when you are seen by different doctors in different clinics. Often, patients arrive at a medical appointment to see a new provider in a new care setting and information is lagging or missing. Or the provider hasn't had time to review the patient chart. Someone has to make sure the system is connected. For instance, if one doctor changes a prescription, you need to tell the other providers of this; or if you have results from a scan, you need to let others know that it was done, why, and the results. Or if you are moving to a new care setting and meeting a new health care provider, you ideally want to summarize your medical history and what happened with your prior care, and what the discharge plans were from the prior setting.

More Than Coordinating Medical Information

It is crucial to integrate the health care system's information with pieces of your personal story and what happens in your private world so that these two realms are not operating as parallel systems. You or your family have the most relevant information about what's happening day to day. You know best what has changed since the last time you saw a health care provider. And you know yourself, your goals, your wishes, and what's happened so far in your illness storyline better than anyone else. Passing along relevant information is a critical role in your team.

For instance, it might be important to tell the doctor that you just lost your brother and you are still grieving; or to explain that your children are really struggling with this diagnosis; or to disclose that you recently lost your job and don't have insurance; or to tell them that you don't have a car and have to catch three buses to get to these appointments. This is critical information that the health system needs to be able to serve you best.

Moreover, someone outside your inner crew won't ever fully appreciate the complexities of integrating the health care world with your private world. For instance, when arranging a home visit, the system likely won't appreciate that you have to take time off work to be present for the home visit. Or when doctors want you to do regular blood work at the hospital, but don't appreciate that it consumes your whole day, as you don't have a car and need to take public transportation. Thus, you or someone in your inner crew always has a role in coordination.

I want to underscore here that while this chapter focuses on the very practical aspects of connecting the dots, the benefits of doing this are far more than just being organized to share information easily. It is a way to maintain a sense of control and to feel more grounded throughout the illness.

All too often, I see patients whose storylines have gotten lost in the chaotic system. They don't feel like themselves anymore. They don't recognize themselves in their journey because there are so many moving parts. They don't have the anchor, which is their story throughout the journey—where they have been up to now. One way to regain that control is to connect the dots. So there is the technical part of managing and organizing information, but there is also the emotional part of seeking meaning between the pieces of information.

Therefore, connecting the dots is also an antidote to the feeling that you have been reduced to pieces and body parts. That you are lost, in the dark, and out of control. That you don't really understand what's happening to you. When you connect the dots, you can retain your sense of control and feel more in charge of where you are heading. You are more connected to your past story, which is important intel to inform your future. You and your family have a front row seat to this intel and have to bring it forward. This is how you can be more activated, empowered, and confident that what you are sharing and asking about is important to your individual illness journey.

Transition Points

We have already described some of the major transition points in an illness, which are

- right after the diagnosis;
- when making decisions about treatment (to start, continue, switch, or stop);
- after any emergency department visit or admission to hospital;
- when transferring between care settings;
- when you notice you are changing (new or worsening symptoms, change in function or ability);
- when making decisions about work (such as considering a leave of absence), place of care, goals of care, or taking a trip;
- when referred to a new care provider; and
- when starting with a new service or support program.

People often assume that these transitions will be well coordinated by the health care system. But transition points are the highest risk times for miscommunication, mistakes with medications, gaps in information, and inconsistent messaging. The danger is that each care team assumes that the other team is taking care of things. Connecting the dots means you are on high alert to prevent important information from falling through the cracks.

Action 1: Identify the Manager

My experience has been that patients who have someone in their inner crew who is the "manager"—someone who is going to keep things organized—have a better illness experience.

You can be the manager. You might be the type of person who likes to take charge and is naturally organized and detail-oriented. Being the manager is a way to remain in the driver's seat of your illness. It might be your style to take the organizer role. In this scenario, it's wise to choose a vice manager, in case there's a time when you get too tired to keep going. The vice manager might also be an extra ear to hear ideas, someone who will share the duties, or a backup.

Not everyone is suited to be a manager. If you prefer to avoid organizing and to take things one day at a time, that's okay. No one is expecting you to change your nature. But then you will need someone in your inner crew who's going to step into the manager role.

I often see that the manager is a spouse or adult offspring. Sometimes two or three people share the role, like siblings caring for an aging parent. But again, it depends on your illness and where you are at in your illness. The manager role does not have to be fixed.

It's worth noting that the manager does not necessarily have to be the primary caregiver. It depends on the situation, the caregiver's natural tendencies and skills, and the caregiver's own health.

The manager's role is also different from a health care proxy, sometimes called the substitute decision maker, though they could be the same person. The health care proxy is legally responsible for making medical decisions on your behalf should you lack the mental capacity to make decisions on your own. To summarize, the manager, caregiver, and health care proxy may be the same person or those roles may be shared by more than one person in your inner crew.

The Manager's Job Description

The manager often takes care of scheduling (and rescheduling) medical appointments or home visits, keeps track of medical information from prior appointments, and calls around and coordinates prescriptions, equipment, and insurance. There is also coordination in your private world, such as who needs to know what information and when and how, and who will do groceries, errands, and childcare while you are receiving medical treatments.

A manager may advocate for you at appointments with health care providers. They should know your style and what is important to you. They keep their finger on the pulse of the appointments, which means they work to untangle the meaning of information provided, research and follow up as needed, and are not afraid to ask questions. They plan ahead by nature. Another key role of the manager is to activate the village, which we talked about in the previous chapter. It is useful, especially if your condition is progressing, to activate people in your various circles of care. Sometimes the manager will create an organizational chart so that it's clear how different tasks (housework, transportation, getting medication, joining medical appointments, scheduling home visits) fall to different members of the inner and outer circles. Having explicit discussions about the roles of different family members can lessen the load on the primary caregiver; it can make the manager's role easier, too.

Finally, besides the doctors and nurses, there are interprofessional care providers (for example, social workers, counselors, physiotherapists, pharmacists, death doulas, and child life specialists) and resources in the community (for example, faith groups, volunteers, and peer support groups) that can be engaged. The role of the manager is to keep track of all the players involved in the formal and informal care team and their roles.

Tip: I recommend defining who will play this role early in your illness. Keeping track of information, juggling schedules, and coordinating details can be overwhelming, especially when someone is thrust into this position later on. When the organization of roles and duties is discussed early in the illness and revisited throughout, it may be easier to manage. It is also important to avoid assigning this vital responsibility to someone who does not want to fulfill the role. If you aren't going to be the manager, ask your preferred person if they will accept the role. You want them to be a prepared guardian of your journey.

EXERCISE: ESTABLISH YOUR MANAGER

A good manager is connected to your inner crew. They should be very organized, able to keep track of lots of moving parts, and competent in clearly and accurately communicating important information between members of the health care team and among the patient and family team members. They are responsible for understanding who needs to know what. Ask yourself:

- Am I going to take on the role of manager (as well as patient)?
- If yes, whom might I choose as my vice manager, in case I need to take a break from the role?

- If not, whom will I ask to be my manager? Is there someone from my inner crew who is already a natural coordinator?

If looking for a manager or vice manager, here are some points to consider:

- Do you trust them?
- Are they capable of making decisions under stress?
- Do they understand your wishes and values?
- Can they communicate clearly to others, including health care providers?
- Are they willing and available?

Action 2: Track Information

It is helpful to create a personal health record that can be shared with the members of the formal health care team. This could be done by the manager or delegated to another person in the inner crew.

At a minimum, it would be helpful for you to track a timeline of the major events of your illness, such as your diagnosis date and when you had major treatments, surgeries, or hospitalizations. It's almost like an illness résumé. It's best to keep it updated in real time when major events occur, in case you need the information later. You don't want to neglect updating it for many years because it will be very hard to go back and remember all the details.

If your condition will progress over time and has the potential to become more complicated and have many moving parts, then you may need to supplement this illness résumé with a more advanced way of keeping track of information—such as your own mini health record. This is especially helpful over time if you are seeing many different clinicians.

This health record can track what's happening in the many hours outside of time with the official health care teams. The health record can be in the form of a diary, journal, notebook, or binder with different tabs. Some patients use mobile apps that they keep on their smartphones. The point is, they are keeping their own notes of what is happening and what is changing in their own patient chart because they know that the different providers in the health care team won't always have the complete picture.

Here are some examples of the types of information you may want to record:

- **Health care team.** Names, role/medical specialty, location
- **Timeline of major medical events.** Treatments received, surgery dates
- **Scan results.** Results and copies of tests, blood work, diagnostic imaging
- **Diary of recent symptoms.** A way to track symptoms over time
- **Equipment.** What type, vendor name, contact info, delivery info
- **Medications.** Prescription names, doses, pharmacy refill info
- **Contacts.** Contact info for key members of the inner crew and your health care teams

There are multiple purposes for this personal record. One is that it might become very important to share among your inner crew. It is also valuable to share among the health care team, especially if many providers are involved, such is often the case with home care services. I have also witnessed that, whether they use the notes or not, people feel more confident when they have all the information tucked away in one area to refer to. It makes them feel more grounded. You will appreciate the entire storyline if you document it and have easy access to it. Finally, anything you can do to organize yourself so that you're not rummaging for important information during a crisis, should one occur, is going to save valuable time.

How detailed you make this personal record will depend on what kind of person you are. It also depends on who is entering the information and keeping it updated over time. Something too onerous is not going to be sustainable. The record can be brief, such as the key highlights in one or two pages, which you add to as critical events happen. Or your notes could be very detailed. Some people document daily symptoms in a diary to track how symptoms are progressing. There isn't a one-size-fits-all method. The key is for the information you track to unite the different parts, people, and health care providers of the system with shared information.

EXERCISE: DECIDE WHAT TO RECORD

Consider what information you want to record and what you hope to do with this information. That will determine how much detail you need and the best way to keep track. Here are some questions to consider:

- Who is going to use this and for what purpose?
- What content do you want to and can you realistically keep track of?
- In what way are you going to keep track of this information (app, journal, notebook, binder, and so on)?
- Who is going to update it?
- How often should it be updated?
- Where will it be kept?
- How will it be shared with other health care providers and/or other family members?

Action 3: Learn about the System You Are In

Learn as much as you can about the health and social systems you have access to, what local resources and services are available to you, what the eligibility criteria are, and how to access them when needed. People will have access to different health care based on geography, service availability, insurance, eligibility, preferences, disease severity, and so on.

A good place to start getting information is from people who have gone through this journey before. They are more likely to give an honest opinion about how coordinated their journey was and the important intel that isn't found in the pamphlets and brochures. Seek out someone who knows what support groups or disease-specific resources are available and helpful, especially if they live in the same area as you.

It's worth noting that you aren't exploring only the supports you need now. At some point, as your condition, needs, or desires change, there may be other supports or services you can benefit from—things you may not know exist. Even though you may not need or be eligible for them now, you may still want to learn about what they offer and how you can access them, so you don't find out about them too late.

Tip: If you need help learning about resources, advocating for support, or processing decisions in a personalized way, a family doctor can be a wonderful resource and sounding board. It's important during the busy stage of many appointments that you don't lose contact with your family doctor. They are a constant along your journey as other specialty teams come and go over time. They may also care for your family members who are experiencing a parallel journey.

EXERCISE: LEARN ABOUT YOUR SYSTEM

You can take multiple steps to equip yourself with invaluable information about the system and resources, and what you need to do for yourself.

- **Seek support:** Investigate peer or support groups for your condition. Consider support groups for you and your family separately, as you may have different needs. Some examples include disease-specific groups by organizations (for example, an Alzheimer's society); community groups and faith groups; online support groups (for example, website forums or Facebook groups). There are also helpful resources that can reduce health care inequities, often found in organizations that specifically serve people who identify as racialized, LGBTQ2IA+, elderly, low income, vulnerably housed, or facing mental health challenges or language barriers.

- **Seek out peers:** Identify people who have your condition or who have cared for someone with your condition. You may find them in a disease support group, as suggested above. You might know someone from your social circles or meet someone in an online forum or the waiting room of the same disease clinic. Arrange to connect and ask them for intel. Ask what their experience was or has been like. What advice or tips do they have? What supports or services were helpful? What equipment was needed? What do they wish they had known sooner?

- **Research:** Learn the rules and regulations about how to access home and community services in your health jurisdiction. These can be publicly funded services or subsidized by your health insurance plans. Learn the eligibility criteria to access these services. Consider researching what private services are available if that's an option for you.

- **Consult with professionals:** Ask health care professionals (for example, your family doctor) about what kinds of services might be helpful for you now and in the future.

Karen's Story: Connecting the Dots

To illustrate this key, I want to share the story of Karen Cumming and her sister. They were loving daughters to their mother, Verna, who had been happily living in an assisted-living facility for four years. One day, Verna woke up and could no longer walk, which meant she had to be moved to a long-term care home or nursing home. Karen told me, "That was the day that our education began." She and her sister had never had any previous education about how the health care system worked. "It was the education of a lifetime. We kept expecting somebody to guide us and to give us the advice we needed," she said. She was shocked to realize that, as she put it, "you better become your own advocates as quickly as possible because no one is there to help you."

I asked her how she knew she had to become the manager of her mother's care. At first, she admitted, she and her sister didn't realize what they had to do. They started every day feeling as if they were drowning. She said, "Our job was just to keep our heads above water. We would wonder, 'What insurmountable issue is going to crop up today? What government bureaucrat do we have to call and wait for a response from? What doctor or nurse do we have to chase to get information from our mother's chart?'" Their overwhelmed feeling came about partly because they didn't do any homework beforehand about how to guide someone into long-term care, and they were unprepared when facing this crisis.

Karen spoke of an early lesson. "All of the medical professionals seemed to be in their own silo," she said. "They were off in their own offices, off in their own worlds. Not only did they not communicate with us very effectively, [but they also] didn't seem to want to communicate with each other." She recalled the pivotal moment when she finally realized that all the health care providers were so busy with their jobs that "they didn't always realize that they could connect with other care coordinators or health care professionals" in charge of Verna's care to provide more efficient and better care. From that moment on, Karen said, "we really understood that if we wanted to make this happen in the best possible way, it was up to us to make it happen."

Karen told me, "One of the best decisions that my sister and I made, very early on, was to buy a very simple spiral-bound notebook at the dollar store." They called it "The Book of Verna." Karen sat down every day in their mother's suite in her assisted-living facility, while Verna was waiting to get into long-term care, and wrote down the details of every conversation with every medical professional who spoke with them. That notebook was their "saving grace." Karen learned that documenting everything that happened was so important because remembering the finer details of every conversation, even the very next day, was a challenge. I also asked her advice for others who had to learn about the system. She encouraged people to "become their own detective and ask great questions... And don't stop until you get the answers you need."

Being an advocate and manager didn't stop for Karen when Verna finally entered a long-term care home. "We had to advocate all over again, just for different things," Karen said. She pointed out that the home itself was a "wonderful place" and the staff were "angelic people," but she had to keep advocating because the health system was chronically understaffed and there weren't enough people to do the job.

This negative experience motivated Karen and her sister to write a book to help others dealing with long-term care. They wanted patients and families "to realize that it is their job to be the project manager of their loved one's care from the very first day, because no one else is going to do it for them." It's too late when you're in the middle of the crisis to then "realize that no one is coming to save you."

Connect the Dots: Summary

- You and your inner crew must connect the different areas of the health care system to your own story inside and outside the hospital walls.
- Choosing a manager for the inner crew is helpful in ensuring continuity of information, especially during transition points. Doing this, you are more likely to feel in control, empowered, safe, and organized.
- Think about where you will record information, who will use it, and how it can be shared. Coordinating across a system is a big job. The more you know about the system you are in, the easier it will be to navigate it.

8

INVITE YOURSELF

“The squeaky wheel gets the oil.”

JOSH BILLINGS

THE KEY Invite Yourself means you can initiate conversations. You do not need to wait for health care providers or family members to broach topics that are on your mind. Doctors often wait for patients and families to lead the conversation so they can follow their lead. This is an opportunity to take control of your experience.

Assumption: Doctors Will Tell Me What I Need to Know, When I Need to Know It

Most people assume that medical professionals are all-knowing. Everyone knows that doctors have gone to school for years to master their craft. Consequently, we trust them implicitly. As a society, we hold them in the highest regard. So when a person has a life-changing diagnosis, they look to their doctor for professional advice.

Patients and their families expect that the doctor will know what to do and when to do it. When a health care provider is dealing with a life-changing illness, it is a familiar call to action, whereas for patients, the diagnosis is usually a first-time experience. Patients and their families wait for their instructions.

They hope that they will have treatment options, and that the doctors will always have another plan. They expect the doctor to keep trying, to come up with the next strategy and continue to magically pull possibilities from their sleeve.

Patients and their families trust that the doctor has good judgment and will help them weigh the benefits and burdens of any decisions. They assume that all options will be presented. When a treatment is offered, the patients and their families often feel a strong sense that they should accept it. After all, why would doctors offer something if they didn't think it was useful?

People put their complete trust in doctors and nurses. The belief is that doctors will tell you what you need to know, when you need to know it. People think that if the doctors are not asking patients questions and not telling them information, then they should just continue to cruise along. They assume that no news is good news. People have faith that their doctor will be truthful, forthcoming, and gentle with information, for better or worse. They also assume doctors know when something bad will occur and will warn them about it. "So as long as I am being offered treatment," they think, "I have ample time. I have nothing to worry about. I have nothing to prepare for now." They refrain from asking the questions that are on their minds. They wait to be invited.

Reality: Doctors Often Wait for You to Initiate Questions

Many doctors feel uncomfortable and tend to avoid inviting patients into open conversations about their illness. Instead, they might default to action-oriented care plans that include more and more treatment. This is because many doctors are not adequately trained, with proper coaching and practice, to have open, honest, and realistic communication with patients and families about all the possibilities, including the options of no treatment or stopping treatment. Even when it is obvious that a person is declining, doctors may offer the next treatment because discussing their limitations to fix or stabilize illness is admitting that doctors are human and that many diseases cannot be cured.

Research suggests that doctors are hesitant to discuss bad news, such as things getting worse, with patients and families because they worry they will cause sadness, anxiety, depression, and hopelessness. They don't want to destroy their patients' hope. They wait for patients or family members to raise the issue, and at the same time, patients and families are waiting for their doctors. The result is that no one is communicating.

Although it is true that some illnesses can be cured, like pneumonia, and some stabilized, like asthma, many others can be neither healed nor halted, like ALS. If the expectation is for the doctor to fix the problem, then when an illness can't be remedied, the doctor may feel helpless. Therefore, instead of gently revealing to the person and family the known reality of the progressive illness, they can be overly optimistic about treatment options, cheerleading for the patient and family to remain hopeful.

The Power Imbalance

Another challenge is that because of power dynamics, patients and families often default to trying to be seen as good and well behaved. They don't want to rock the boat or cause issues or complain too much. They fear that the doctor-patient relationship or the care provided might be altered or worsened if they are labeled difficult. Some people are so focused on being good patients that they end up becoming passive. They hesitate to ask questions because they don't want to sound silly or waste the doctor's precious time. They hesitate to offer information for the same reason.

But doctors and nurses assume that if patients and families want more information, they'll ask. They also assume that if there is something important to know, the patients or families will tell them. Here we have two sides: the patients being polite and good and the medical professionals assuming that they have no questions.

The Communication Vacuum

Unfortunately, passive patients and families are at the mercy of the health care system. As time goes on, the illness journey becomes busier. When this pattern of the "passive patient–busy clinician" dynamic is set in motion, a huge gap forms, where no one is communicating on either side. The elephant in the room is growing. The doctor, patient, and family are easily distracted into tangential discussions. A communication vacuum forms. This can be dangerous.

What I see in my patients with a progressive, life-limiting condition is that they put unwavering trust in their health care providers. The patient and family start wondering what is happening, but they take their cues from the doctor. This leads to being steered toward treatment-favored care for too long. Too often, the patient does not fully understand that their condition is a progressive, life-limiting condition. And then at some late point in time, when they are told there is nothing more that can be done, they feel abandoned. They feel like it's a sudden drop off a cliff.

Patricia's Story: In the Dark

When I met Patricia, her husband, Larry, was seventy-nine and undergoing treatment for stage 4 lung cancer. He had already lived four years since his diagnosis. He was now on his second line of immunotherapy, which means he had already gone through the regular cycles of treatment, and after that stopped working, they were on to another type of treatment, which would be less effective than the first. Patricia was very worried about what was going to happen after this line of treatment ended. She knew there would be a day when it would not work anymore. Larry was already getting a bit weaker from his treatments. She confided in me that she was very worried about how she was going to pay for treatment after this line of immunotherapy ended. When I asked her if she had talked with the oncologist, she said, "I can't ask. She's so busy. Also, every time we go to the clinic, she tells us how great he looks and how well we are doing on the treatment. I guess we are doing better than most of her patients, so I don't want to waste her time with unnecessary questions."

As a patient, Larry had the right to ask questions and receive answers, though he was happy to just live day to day. But Patricia also had the right to voice her questions and concerns, especially as the primary caregiver. As the manager, she was trying to think ahead and be proactive. But she was ultimately afraid to invite herself to the conversation because she felt the spotlight should be on Larry, and she did not want to take away his hope. But this left her with unanswered questions and unmet needs.

Consequences. When communication lines are closed, families and patients are left with whatever is shared with them, which might not be the information they need to plan ahead. Open conversations about the future get kicked down the road. Without the answers they need, people can feel anxious and scared, and these types of emotions can amplify physical symptoms. And this becomes a vicious cycle. They start feeling more physical symptoms, which makes them more worried and anxious.

Claire's Story: In the Know

I want to share the story of Claire Snyman, a brain tumor survivor, brain injury patient and advocate, and author. She was thirty-four, a wife and a mother of a four-year-old son, living her life, when one day she suddenly had a vertigo spell, followed by migraines lasting for a few days. She eventually went to the emergency department, where she learned that she had a rare, non-malignant brain tumor. She was put under a watch-and-wait plan that did not require surgery or treatment yet.

Claire went from being a normal person to being someone who "now had multiple medications, multiple appointments, multiple MRI scans and tests, and multiple specialists." She had to quickly learn how to navigate the health care system and be active in monitoring her symptoms and care. She kept copies of all the MRIs she had year after year for her own records. She previously hadn't appreciated the "rather tumultuous sort of navigation of the health care system" that patients go through routinely.

Claire said, "[I realized I had to] surround myself with a solid and robust medical team that were able to give me the best and most accurate sort of care that I needed. And I did that. I even got a second opinion to make sure that I had the right diagnosis and the right treatment and way forward. And that made me feel the most secure about what was happening to me with my treatments and [gave me] a way forward. And that made me feel less uncertain."

This was important because after two years, her brain tumor had doubled in size and blocked the flow of the fluid in her brain, causing her brain to swell. This required emergency brain surgery, which also led to a long-lasting brain injury.

Her ability to invite herself to her care early on involved implementing what she calls the TEAM approach:

- Track everything
- Educate yourself
- Ask questions
- Manage your health care

She also had to seek information, including knowing the type of symptoms she should look for that might indicate the tumor was growing. But Claire also had to seek hidden information about the "mental health challenges that could affect an individual who had a brain tumor" and that would appear long after surgery.

She also recognized early on that her husband had to have a key role in her care, especially because she had a brain injury. "He was integral in knowing my health care, my patterns at home, everything like that." He had critical insight because sometimes the impacts of brain injury are not immediately evident to others—it's an invisible disability. Her husband knew all of the intricacies of Claire's usual patterns and the details of her condition.

Inviting yourself is about being an activated patient. Claire said, "I really needed to step up and get involved. A medical error and misdiagnosis happened just before my surgery. And if I hadn't been an activated patient, we wouldn't be having this conversation today."

Benefits. The only way to be prepared and aware is to seek information. And the only way to make the journey personalized is to share. Doing this is meant to protect you from feeling silenced, ignored, or in the dark, all of which amplifies suffering. Inviting yourself can lead to more optimal treatment, more coordinated care—a smoother journey. But it can also prevent medical errors and mistakes because you are an active participant in your care plan and decisions.

How to Invite Yourself

Invite Yourself might be the most powerful key in the book because all the other keys require you to invite yourself and speak up. You need to keep information flowing and not wait for it to come your way. It's an active skill to share, invite, role-model, seek, and ask. This key is about finding your voice, being brave, and getting activated.

Fundamentally, inviting yourself is about two-way communication: asking questions and sharing information. Doctors have vital medical information you may want to seek out; you and your family have vital information that is important to share, such as your worries, concerns, sense of your family's coping, noticing changes in your daily routines, and so on. You're not there to passively receive information. You have a key role to bring forward your insights.

This key is ultimately about taking back control of your illness experience. You don't need permission to start a conversation with your health care providers or your inner crew, or to ask questions that are important to you. Knowledge is power. Information is power. It is grounding.

Inviting yourself is about moving from the back seat of your illness, where you are a passive passenger, to the front seat with a clear view of what's ahead. You can drive for yourself or let someone you trust be the driver, but you want to at least be in the front seat to navigate the route.

The earlier you do it, and the more often you do it, the more in the know and prepared you will be. Especially for illnesses that will change over time, it's helpful to be aware and to prepare for future twists and turns and the multiple decisions that arise along the journey.

There may be times when you don't like the answers you get. You may receive news you did not expect or want to hear. You might feel overwhelmed or scared or sad. But like the majority of people I meet, after you have some time to digest the news, you will feel better, more in control, and more grounded. You are more resilient than you might give yourself credit for. And you will be able to move forward and make better decisions when you have all the information.

Being Respectfully Assertive

Sometimes, in a busy clinic, you might feel like there's no time or opportunity to ask questions or, if you ask something, you are quickly shut down. This is when you have to not only invite yourself but also be respectfully assertive.

My experience is that patients and family members who assert themselves are more likely to get the information they need. Sometimes this means advocating for something. Often, speaking up is asking questions, seeking information, and being direct and clear. It's as the saying goes: "The squeaky wheel gets the oil." That said, this is not suggesting you be rude or disrespectful. There are many ways to be direct and assertive while being respectful and civil.

Speak up to *seek* information when

- you have a doubt,
- you need clarification,
- you have a concern or worry, or
- you notice a change in your condition.

Speak up to *offer* information when

- you transition from one health care setting to another,
- you meet new health care providers and you need to share your history,
- you feel that key information is missing or not being considered, or
- you notice a change in your condition.

Tip: If speaking up or using conversation starters seems too uncomfortable, consider inviting someone else to join you in these appointments. Often, it's more comfortable to speak up when you have someone by your side. Most people benefit from having a companion at appointments, someone to provide moral support, take notes, ask pointed questions, and seek clarification if you feel too shy or drained to do this on your own. It's especially helpful to buddy up with someone who isn't afraid to speak up if being assertive is not your natural style.

Inviting Your Loved Ones In

In my experience, patients sometimes try to shield their family from their illness experience to protect them. But the end result is that family members become more conflicted: they want to understand what is happening, how to plan and prepare, how to get ready for whatever is ahead. But when they are being shielded, they feel helpless. And they stay quiet because they haven't been invited into the fold by you, the person with the illness.

A charade develops with both patient and family doing an awkward dance around open, honest communication with each other. The atmosphere becomes polite, superficial, and devoid of any real conversation about the illness experience. Loved ones adopt a cheerleader role because they have no permission to be real, even when they want to be.

I gently encourage you to give your family or inner crew full permission to initiate questions at the beginning, middle, late, and end stages of your illness. They should be fully aware of what this illness entails so they can meet your needs as well as their own. The more they know, the more they can prepare for what lies ahead and advocate with you and for you.

Family Shout-Out: Family members, especially the primary caregiver, must know how to advocate for themselves and the patient, too. The family caregivers are often isolated from interactions with the health care providers. They might be ignored at appointments, where the focus is on the patient. Families often tell me they feel invisible or ignored. They also feel conflicted about contributing their observations because they don't want to betray the positive vibe or divulge information that has not been previously discussed with the patient. They sit in the room beside their loved one and take on a passive role. Many family members resent that they are never given the chance to meet with the health care clinicians alone. They just go with the flow and keep their insights and worries to themselves. The consequences of the family caregivers waiting to be invited include resentment, stress, burden, fatigue, and confusion.

I always encourage primary caregivers to heed the practical actions of this key—Invite Yourself—such as asking and sharing. Ask questions to be in the know and share the information you have, since you have the best sense of how the patient is doing in between doctor visits. In fact, you can share information with the health care team even when the patient is not there, such as in a phone call. However, in most places, health care providers cannot give you information about the patient without the patient's explicit consent.

Fear of Being Labeled Difficult

One of the biggest challenges of inviting yourself is the fear of being labeled difficult and getting sub-optimal care. While the potential of being labeled difficult might be hard to accept, and it is not fair or appropriate, you should not be quieted by it, either. Take courage in the fact that you and your family know things that no health care professional would ever be expected to know. So it's important that you feel confident enough to bring this information forward. Again, you are the expert in you; they are the expert in treating the illness.

Julie Drury, a caregiver mother, told me of the helpful mindset she kept when she was advocating for her sick daughter in the hospital every day: be "gently fierce." She explained that this attitude encouraged her to not let her voice be silent and to insist that she be included. She told me she "makes no apologies for being relentless" and finding answers to her questions. "You cannot wait for the system to come to you," Julie said. "You need to go to the system." The key to this approach is to treat health care providers with kindness and humility, reminding yourself that most of them want to help their patients in the best ways possible.

It's worth noting that for some people, and in some cultures and marginalized groups, not "rocking the boat" and avoiding being a "squeaky wheel" are learned coping strategies. If this is true for you too, I especially encourage you to consider what Invite Yourself would mean for you. And to develop strategies so that your voice can be respectfully brought forward and your preferences advocated for. There are unconscious biases in the health care system that more quickly label patients as "difficult" due to language and cultural differences. However, this is not the time to be silent.

Tip: Here are some ways to be respectful of the health care provider's time:

- Do your own research, as best you can.
- Prioritize your questions. Write them down.
- At the beginning of the appointment, indicate that you have a number of burning questions to ask at some point before the appointment ends.
- Make a separate and potentially longer appointment to answer your questions if you run out of time.

EXERCISE: REFLECT ON FEAR

Here are some of the common fears that prevent patients from inviting themselves and some potential ways to address them. See if any apply to you.

Fear: My natural style is not assertive; I tend to be shy or a peacekeeper. I don't like conflict.

Consider this: Buddy up with someone in your inner crew who is comfortable speaking up on your behalf.

Fear: I am worried about wasting my doctor's time. I don't want to appear to be asking silly questions.

Consider this: Asking questions is positive. It shows that you are engaged and want to be proactive. Often, doctors are waiting for you to ask before talking more about important topics.

Fear: I'm afraid that I'll be labeled a problematic patient and this will lead to not getting the best care.

Consider this: Be gently fierce. You can ask questions or point out issues in direct, clear ways while remaining respectful. Don't worry too much about being "labeled"—this is your care; this is your life. You have to advocate for yourself.

Fear: I want to be a good patient. I don't want to disappoint my doctors.

Consider this: Your doctors are there to provide care that is best for you. If you don't invite yourself, they won't know how to customize their care to what is important to you.

Action 1: Seek and Share

We have already discussed different ways to check in at key transition points of your illness when there are choices or decisions to be made. Here are some questions you should ask yourself, your family, or your care team:

- Where am I at in this illness (i.e., beginning, middle, late, or end stage)?
- What will this next phase look like?
- What are the kinds of things my family and I need to get ready for?
- What have I learned so far in my illness?
- What do I value?
- What am I most worried about?

Saving up a lot of unanswered questions and trying to get them all answered in one visit is not ideal. Your doctor will probably run out of time. Ask and share throughout the illness journey—whatever is on your mind, so you can start preparing and being proactive. You can invite yourself to ask questions. Small, medium, and large. Anything on your mind is fair game.

You are also invited to share important details about yourself with providers and your inner crew. Here are some examples:

- How you like to hope for the best, but want to plan for the rest (Walk Two Roads)
- Your understanding of the big picture of your illness and where you think you are at (Zoom Out)

- How much information you want and how you like to get information and cope (Know Your Style)
- Your goals or hopes, or practical things like finances or insurance (Customize Your Order)
- Who your inner crew is and your manager (Anticipate Ripple Effects)
- Any information learned from other providers that you are bringing to this appointment (Connect the Dots)

Being proactive also involves making plans to stay ahead of potential hurdles. Here are some examples of questions to consider for yourself, your family, and/or your health care team:

- What action plan can we put in place if I end up having a severe symptom down the road?
- What action plan can we put in place if I have a seizure or fall?
- What action plan can we put in place if I am no longer able to get to my bathroom in my home?

It's extremely important to think ahead and create action plans for common situations that people with your illness are likely to experience. You don't want to develop the action plan when a crisis happens. By then, it's too late.

Action 2: Renew Your Vows

To help you understand each of your health care providers' roles in your care, early on in the illness you should think about clarifying and/or reaffirming their commitment to your ongoing care. I call this "renewing your vows" because it reminds me of when life partners renew their vows with each other after being together for a long time. Similarly, you can sit down with your health care providers and teams, especially your primary care provider, and renew your vows together. Find out if and how they will be there for you as your needs change and your illness progresses.

Renewing your vows early in the illness trajectory, even after a diagnosis, opens up the communication channels and strengthens the trust between you and the clinicians. It elicits and clarifies your goals of care, gets pertinent information early, and encourages ongoing conversations about the complexity and uncertainty of your illness in your future. A one-time conversation is never adequate to prepare patients. You need ongoing support and preparation about what to expect because, as I've mentioned, things change over the course of an illness.

Regardless of who you renew your vows with, be it your primary care provider or specialist, there are a few things you should consider: how well and for how long you have known the provider, what your relationship is like, and how well they know your inner crew and caregivers. This information will help you determine the nature of the conversation, the types of questions you will ask, and whether you want them to be a part of your core team for the rest of your illness.

Primary Care Provider

Depending on your situation, you probably had a home base for your care before you got your life-changing diagnosis. For most people, that is a family doctor (sometimes called a general practitioner or primary care provider), nurse practitioner, or medical clinic. Many people have known their primary care provider for many years, though over the course of an illness, they typically see them less and less—sometimes not at all for years—as they are followed by their disease-specific specialist. But your primary care provider is often responsible for your overarching health. They can play a critical role in the continuity of care and information and also in customizing the care plan to fit what's important to you.

Conversation Starters: When renewing your vows, ask your primary care provider:

- "Are you willing to recommit to staying involved in my care throughout the illness journey, for better or worse?"
- "Do you care for your patients across their entire lifespan?"
- "How will you care for me across the illness trajectory? How do you manage if your patients begin to decline?"
- "What things can you help me with or offer me at different stages?"
- "How comfortable are you with speaking openly about the long view of the illness?" (Declare your preference for how open you would like them to be.)

You may also want to ask:

- "Which health care providers, including from other disciplines (social worker, pharmacists, spiritual counselor, dietician, and so on), are part of your practice?"
- "How does your practice work with and communicate with my other specialists?"
- "How can we stay in an efficient communication loop?" (For example, who should I call for what issue? And how do I share information if I notice changes in my condition?)

You may also want to explain to your primary care provider who your main caregivers are so they may all talk about your care, and any other needs, directly. If you don't have a primary care doctor, you might consider getting one or a place that will become your medical home for your ongoing needs.

Specialists

When you are dealing with a life-changing illness, it is common to be referred to a disease specialist. I call these the "ologists": there's the cardiologist, respirologist, oncologist, nephrologist, and so on. The specialist's disease expertise becomes the focus of medical appointments, sometimes for many years.

Again, if your illness changes and progresses over time, the core team you deal with may shift. Sometimes this shift is overt ("we are transferring you back to your family doctor now" or "you can follow up with your family doctor now"), and sometimes it is not clear ("there is no need to book any more follow-up visits with us"). So, clarifying what your specialist team is (and isn't) responsible for is important. This is a variation of renewing your vows with disease specialists.

Conversation Starters: Here are some examples of things to ask your disease specialist when you renew your vows with them:

- "When an emergency happens, whom should I call?"
- "Whom do I call if I have a symptom issue or important question?"
- "Do you have other members of your specialist team, such as nurses or coordinators? Who on your team is responsible for what?"
- "What is your role in my illness? In what situation does the responsibility get passed on to someone else?"

Action 3: Start Proactive Practices Now

Especially if your illness is progressive and life-limiting, you may want to be more intentional and proactive with your main health care provider, such as your family doctor. You have to switch gears from "no news is good news" or going to the doctor only when you have a major issue.

You and your family need to remain vigilant throughout your illness to *revisit* the big picture with your health care team. Requesting regular check-ins with the doctors and inviting ongoing discussion about the big picture of the illness will lead to more coordinated care. For instance, ask if you can proactively book follow-up check-in appointments. These check-in visits help you keep track of your illness over time. This longitudinal relationship and continuity of care will allow your health care provider to better pick up on subtle changes in your condition.

Regular visits with your health care provider will also make it easier for you to bring up emerging concerns before they become major issues. Depending on your condition and how quickly you and your doctor understand things might change, you can book appointments with them every week, month, or every two to six months.

You might also ask if you need longer visits sometimes. Here you can go more into depth talking about possible hurdles and discuss action plans. For example, before the need arises, ask if your family doctor does home visits.

Conversation Starters: Here are examples of questions to ask your family doctor that support proactive care practices:

- "Can we schedule regular check-in appointments, as appropriate, to discuss expected changes in the illness?"
- "Do you offer telephone support?"
- "Do you make home visits, if required?"
- "When more time is needed, can you offer longer appointments or book me in the first or last appointment of the day?"
- "What is your after-hours or on-call availability?"
- "What resources and supports are available?" (For example, caregiver support groups, financial benefits, or options for private care.)

Donna's Story: Invite Yourself

To illustrate this key, I want to share an interview I did with Donna Thomson, caregiver advocate and author. Donna's life completely changed when her son Nicholas was born with cerebral palsy, along with many other complex conditions, including being nonverbal from birth. A former actor and teacher, Donna became the primary caregiver of her very medically complex son. Donna's journey has led her to become a vocal caregiving and disability advocate and author.

At the time of this writing, Nicholas is a thirty-four-year-old "living his best adult life" in a medical group home with one-to-one twenty-four-hour awake nursing care. But when he was young, he was hospitalized with many different childhood illnesses. Without exaggeration, he has had ninety-nine hospitalizations in his life to date, including major surgeries to try to correct things like a dislocated hip. All the interventions they pursued for his orthopedic issues had negative, unintended outcomes, resulting in chronic and acute pain that he has to this day.

Donna acknowledged that she experienced the "egos [of providers] and the hierarchies of power in health care," which left her at times feeling like she was "being punished" for advocating for something that was contrary to what members of the health care team recommended. There were many instances when she had to advocate for Nicholas and speak for him, since he is nonverbal. I asked if this led her to being labeled "difficult" and she flat-out said yes. But she added: "This is not the time to be quiet, because it's just too important. There's just too much at stake to really make assumptions."

It resonated with her that "clinicians, by default, are not going to want to make you sad, are not going to want to potentially enter a messy exchange with emotions." She said she thought that they were having honest conversations, but they weren't. Her advice now is to "explicitly give permission to [health care providers] to be honest. And say, 'This is the conversation that I want and this is what I need.'"

For instance, there was a major disconnect between what the doctors were saying and what she was understanding. Donna recollected: "We know now that he cannot sit in his chair for more than an hour and a half at a time. But in those days, I wanted him to go back to the disabled ski program. I wanted him to have his active life that he had before his hip problems. And I was on a mission to get them to fix him so that he could be active. And they did not want to tell me that that was not possible. What they told me was: 'You need to adjust his lifestyle.' They wouldn't tell me, 'His active life is over.'" There were a "multitude of unanswered questions and a multitude of incorrect assumptions on my part. And nobody to talk to about what any of this meant for Nicholas, for me, and for our family."

Donna stressed the importance of seeking and sharing. She wished she had asked more questions. She wished she had shared more about her goals for Nicholas. For instance, there was a time when she believed "that if [they] just worked harder, tried more things, that Nicholas could have a set active life back." This goal sharing would have allowed her health care team an opening to explain which goals were realistic and which were not.

Renewing the vows and proactive practices were critical for Donna when Nicholas was older and needed to move from pediatric care to adult care. At that time, they needed to find a family doctor who would take on a complex patient. They needed to determine upfront the people involved in Nicholas's circle of care (including nurses who were providing round-the-clock care in their home), and what each person's role would be, including the family doctor. For instance, was he willing to make home visits? (The answer was yes.) The proactive practices included using an online medical care coordination tool so Nicholas's medical records and notes could be shared across health care providers and the family. They had to negotiate who would be the one to call if there was an emergency, what constituted an emergency, and how they would communicate in a timely manner.

Donna's final advice to new patients was, "Do not assume anything." Ask questions if you aren't sure, and share your understanding and goals to create the opportunity to clarify misunderstandings. She added that the practice of inviting yourself "is absolutely key to having any degree of success in going through a health challenge."

Invite Yourself: Summary

- Don't wait for doctors to invite you to the conversation. You can initiate the conversations you want to have. Be gently fierce. This will allow you to take back some of the control that illness takes from you.
- Seek and share information, role modeling the kind of communication and proactive approach that you want throughout the illness.
- Consider renewing your vows with your family doctor and explore implementing proactive practices with them.

All of this also applies to family caregivers, who are often invisible to the health system.

9

PUTTING IT ALL TOGETHER

"If you learn a recipe,
you can cook the recipe.
If you learn the technique,
you can cook anything."

MICHAEL SYMON

THE SEVEN KEYS to being hopeful and prepared were born from the experiences of thousands of patients and families before you who told me, "I wish I'd known that sooner." Many shared their stories hoping to benefit future patients, such as you. The keys represent the skills common among those who had a better illness experience.

Assumption: The Keys Should Be Used in Order

Because I have numbered the keys, you might assume that they are steps to be applied in order, from Walk Two Roads onward, and that you have to enact each key successfully before proceeding to the next one, like following steps in a recipe. Or you might assume that the early keys are more relevant for the beginning and middle stages of an illness, and the latter keys are used for the end stage of the illness storyline.

Reality: The Keys Can Be Blended Together

The seven keys are not steps or stages that follow a particular order but are instead fluid. They are meant to be blended together and used as needed to help you be in the know. The keys can be used at different times and in different combinations. Once you are aware of them, you can incorporate them into the way you walk your entire journey.

How to Put It All Together

I have now revealed each of the seven keys to navigating a life-changing diagnosis:

- Walk Two Roads
- Zoom Out
- Know Your Style
- Customize Your Order
- Anticipate Ripple Effects
- Connect the Dots
- Invite Yourself

How you use and blend these keys together will depend greatly on your illness, its trajectory, and your circumstances. For instance, you might be naturally assertive, so you already practice Invite Yourself, but you may need support to Anticipate Ripple Effects and Customize Your Order. Another example is that you might only need to Connect the Dots if multiple providers get involved or system navigation gets complicated. Everyone is different.

That said, Walk Two Roads is the gateway skill. You need to start with being open to exploring the what-ifs before you can prepare for what is to come. Once you are aware of the other road, you can zoom out and obtain truthful information about the big picture of your illness. The other skills follow.

These keys are not meant to put more stress on you, though it may feel overwhelming to enact all that I have suggested. But I've seen over and over that if you take them up, you are more likely to avoid ending up in the dark and going deeper into it at each new chapter of the illness. Although activating the keys right now might seem like a huge task, you may be surprised by how natural they become. It's like learning a new language. It's hard at first, but with practice, you feel more fluent.

My goal in sharing the seven keys is to allow you to reclaim your role as the driver of your health care journey, rather than taking the default role, which often feels like being a passive passenger in the back seat. Using the skills will increase your sense of self; they will give you more agency in enacting your preferences. I hope they transform the way you interact with your family and health care providers.

I also hope the information I have offered transforms the kind of patient you are so that, to the extent you want, you are fully informed about and actively involved in the decisions along your care journey. So that you can move from being in the dark to fully in the know.

Special Considerations

This is not a one-size-fits-all approach. Unique populations require additional care and considerations, as they have historically been underserved and marginalized. They may encounter barriers and resistance in trying to obtain information and appropriate care.

This book does not fully address the unique challenges of each of these populations, which are sufficiently diverse groups themselves. There are likely resources specific to each population or group that complement the seven skills. Nonetheless, these skills can help address some of the systemic barriers and false assumptions that exist. Let's briefly look at some unique populations and the keys that may have additional relevance.

Racialized Communities

Because of systemic racism, people from racialized communities, such as those who identify as BIPOC (Black, Indigenous, People of Color), may face additional overt or hidden barriers to accessing or receiving optimal care. There is often a long history of mistrust in the hierarchy and power structures of the health system, which are biased toward a Western, colonial, biomedical perspective. For support in addressing such barriers, think about who in your community might have already walked this road and who may have advice to offer. I encourage you to identify culturally safe support agencies in your area or online that might have different resources to help you navigate the system in a way that respects your racial and ethnic background (Connect the Dots).

It is critical to not be lulled into simply following the doctor's orders without question; try to bring forward what is important to you and who you are as a person, including any cultural or spiritual beliefs (Customize Your Order). This is important to do as early and safely as you can in your journey, not only during critical medical decisions, as it enables your health care providers to understand who you are fully. The way certain cultures talk about illness or dying, who and how they care for and make decisions about the sick, and where care occurs all are influenced, in part, by the cultures people were raised in. With this knowledge, based on what you share, providers might approach conversations and information-sharing differently. They can also flag opportunities for you to adapt standard protocols to better match your preferences. For instance, for some of my patients, personal autonomy and privacy are paramount, whereas for others, the entire family is heavily involved in decision-making. Some patients prefer to pass away at home; others, in a hospital. Therefore, sharing your beliefs and experiences early can have positive ripple effects.

LGBTQ2IA+ Communities

LGBTQ2IA+ people may face additional barriers in the health care system. If you identify as part of this community, you may encounter heterosexism, homophobia, or transphobia, and may be faced with the decision about whether or not to come out to your health care providers and to each new team of specialists you deal with (Invite Yourself). Because different jurisdictions have different legal parameters around recognizing LGBTQ2IA+ rights, you may need to do due diligence to ensure that legal aspects of your care and decision-making are respected. For instance, if you have a long-term partner but are not legally wed to them, you may experience challenges in some jurisdictions where partners are not automatically legally recognized as substitute decision makers and thus have no rights as to proxy medical decision-making. If they are not automatically recognized, it is worth exploring ways in which you can name your desired health care proxy (Customize Your Order). If strained family dynamics are part of the situation, it will be important for you to declare who your inner crew is to the health care team, so they know who should and should not receive your medical information (Anticipate Ripple Effects). You may need to look for agencies and resources that are specific to supporting LGBTQ2IA+ communities (Connect the Dots).

The system is far from perfect, however. Gaps in care for racialized and LGBTQ2IA+ communities are well documented. This may mean that skillful advocacy, communication, and self-care for you and your family are particularly important.

Patients Experiencing Language Barriers

If you cannot communicate with your health care providers because you speak a different language, medical translators can be helpful and may need to be organized ahead of time (Connect the Dots). Having a trusted family member or friend who can translate during the visits will be helpful (Anticipate Ripple Effects). Even if the person cannot be available for every health care appointment, prioritize booking a translator for an early appointment, where the goal is to ascertain the big picture of the illness and where you are in that trajectory.

Patients Who Live Alone or Have Remote Caregivers

For this population, there is more pressure on the patient to take initiative and to explore the resources in their area (Connect the Dots). As you now know, it is important to identify who, if anyone, forms your inner crew, such as neighbors, children, friends, or other (paid or unpaid) care providers (Anticipate Ripple Effects). Otherwise, you ought to consider contingency plans, such as moving to a place with additional health care support if that is required. Remote caregivers, who are likely in the second ring of support because of geography, can still play a role, such as employing remote monitoring technology, hiring help, investigating resources online or by phone, and so on. Understanding the expected next stages of an illness is critical (Zoom Out). Your knowledge of this can inform proactive planning—for example, understanding your eligibility criteria for supportive services or getting added to a wait list for an alternate place of care, like a hospice.

When the Patient Is a Child

When children are sick, there is enormous pressure to stay exclusively on the road of hope. It can feel much harder to hope for the best but plan for the rest (Walk Two Roads). There are professionals such as child life specialists or social workers who have specific training in working with juvenile patients and their families. Understanding the big picture of the illness is critical to assess whether any changes are just one-offs or a sign of moving to another stage in the illness (Zoom Out). Child patients, especially teenagers, often develop a sense of their values and goals over time. It may be difficult for parents, but trying to listen to understand the patient's priorities and what they value most is vital for informed decision-making throughout the illness (Customize Your Order).

Patients with Housing or Food Insecurity

Some regions have health resources for unhoused and low-income patients, and it is worthwhile researching what may be available to you if you fall in this category (Connect the Dots). Also, do not assume that clinicians understand your priorities (Customize Your Order). For instance, any health care recommendations have to be considered in the context of available shelter and meals. As in any situation, declare who your inner crew is to your health care team, whether those are shelter coordinators, friends, family, or chosen family, so they know whom to share medical information with and who you want as your health care proxy (Anticipate Ripple Effects).

Dealing With Resistance

Whatever your background and life situation, you will surely meet some resistance in the health care system as you assert your needs. In fact, it is one of the most common frustrations I hear from patients and families: they feel as though their doctors aren't listening or responding to their questions. My advice is to persist.

I find it is helpful to say to your provider that you recognize they are very busy and you would therefore like to request a longer appointment or family meeting to go through the important questions you and your family have (Anticipate Ripple Effects). This is a great opportunity for a conversation to understand the big picture of your illness (Zoom Out) or to renew your vows (Invite Yourself).

I also suggest bringing someone with you to appointments to help advocate for you, prioritizing your questions ahead of time (Invite Yourself), and sharing your information-seeking style (Know Your Style). It is also worthwhile to explain to your health care providers the motivation behind why you are seeking more information (Customize Your Order), such as your desire to be grounded in open and realistic information (Walk Two Roads).

If you do meet resistance, remember that this experience is only one encounter, the resistance perhaps from a singular health care provider. If one particular provider keeps avoiding your questions, you can try asking other members of your health care team. Health care providers are as unique and different as patients and families. I know lots of doctors and nurses who are just waiting for an invitation to speak openly to their patients and families. Also, be mindful that you are proceeding as an activated patient before the health care system has had time to adjust. The first time you bring up your questions, health care providers might be unsure how to answer some of them. It's a process. It takes practice.

But if you keep asking and are persistent, they will hopefully return next time with better answers. You're planting seeds, and you need to keep watering them throughout the journey. You are role modeling the type of care you want. The type of patient you are now. The way you want information provided to you. Information is power.

It's a process for you, too. Remember to be gentle on yourself. You might also need some practice. It takes bravery and courage. You will develop your own way to enact the keys, one that feels comfortable to you, and your own way of phrasing things, so it fits with your style. Remember, you are uniquely positioned to enact the keys, customize your experience, and take charge of your illness journey.

So far, the seven keys we've presented are for anyone facing a life-changing diagnosis, whether it's chronic, progressive, and/or life-limiting. However, the next two chapters are written specifically for people who have a life-limiting illness. These chapters describe in more detail the late and end stages of an illness. In chapter 10, I describe how to identify the tipping point that begins the final decline in an illness, which is typically sometime in the last year of life. In chapter 11, I discuss some of the biggest myths related to dying that can cause unnecessary anxiety and fears.

You can choose whether or not to read the next two chapters. Think about sharing these final chapters with someone in your inner crew. As I have mentioned before, information is empowering. There is nothing worse than catastrophizing dying. Overwhelmingly, my patients and their families feel so thankful when we invite open, honest, truthful information about dying. Many say to me, "I feel so much better now that I know."

Putting It All Together: Summary

- The keys are not meant to be used in order, but rather blended together. Every person is unique and the keys will need to be applied differently according to your circumstances or as is relevant throughout your illness.
- Unique populations, especially underserved and marginalized people, will require additional care and consideration. There are supports that serve diverse populations that should be sought out early.
- You will likely meet resistance. Stay persistent over the entire journey.

10

WHEN TIME IS RUNNING OUT

“Lost time is
never found again.”

BENJAMIN FRANKLIN

EVERY PROGRESSIVE, life-limiting illness has a beginning, middle, late, and end stage. I often say that when patients reach the late stage of an illness, which is approximately the last year of life, they are at the tipping point.

Assumption: Dying Comes Suddenly

Most people assume they will die rather suddenly. I have met so many patients who were scared to close their eyes at night because they were worried they'd never open them again, as if they would suddenly die without notice or warning. Many of my patients feel that dying is like turning off a light switch.

Reality: Dying Happens Over Time

The reality is that only 10 percent of us will die an unexpected, sudden death. The remaining 90 percent will die of a progressive, chronic illness or from frailty in old age. Although progressive illnesses each have their unique trajectory with ups and downs, the tipping point typically doesn't occur suddenly.

The final descent usually happens slowly, over a year or months. Most people fade over time, and you can see it coming. Therefore, for the vast majority of us, dying should feel more like a light dimmer.

But too many resist acknowledging the transition to the advanced stage of illness despite the fact there are clear physical signs when our time is running out. The early signs of dying are often subtle, rationalized as due to other causes, brushed under the carpet, or lost in the pursuit of tests and treatments. A patient may be deteriorating but not realize they are beginning to die until the very end of their life.

Even though death is an expected outcome for everyone with a progressive, life-limiting illness, most people have no idea of what to expect for this final chapter. We prepare for every other life event, from birth to graduation to marriage to retirement. Yet a road map for the dying phase of a life-limiting illness is hard to find. This is because as a society, we are conditioned to not only deny the possibility that we will die but also fear it so badly that we do not let our minds wander that far into the future. It feels scary. To manage this fear, people will take things one day at a time. This can leave them unprepared, reactive, and crisis-driven. When the end comes, it is seen as sudden instead of expected. But a progressive, non-curable illness usually enters into the dying phase sometime between months and a year before death.

Neil's Story: In the Dark

I met Neil, a man with cancer, a handful of weeks before he died. I was asked to see him in his home because he was experiencing unrelenting nausea and vomiting, along with fatigue and low energy. The assumption was that it was likely caused by his chemotherapy. The oncologist suggested a compromise: that he continue his treatment at half the strength. But Neil's symptoms did not improve.

I had a difficult discussion with Neil, sharing with him that one option was to stop the chemotherapy altogether so his symptoms would abate. Neil was shocked when I pointed out that his fatigue and low energy weren't just about the side effects of his treatment—he had started down the road of decline. His body was succumbing to the cancer, and he would continue to lose stamina until the end, even if he stayed on the chemotherapy. "Well, why the hell didn't someone tell me this earlier?" he asked, as if he suddenly felt scammed by other health care providers. "Wow, I would have stopped this chemotherapy months ago had someone bothered to tell me that I was deteriorating. I just assumed that my low energy was a side effect of the treatment."

In his final weeks, he continued down a slippery slope. This was hardly an ideal time to suddenly settle all of his affairs. His house was jam-packed with personal items. Nothing was organized and sorted. He didn't have funeral arrangements or a will. This unfinished business worried Neil more than his condition and contributed to his anxiety and distress in the ensuing weeks. The only thing he managed to do was have his brother come to listen to his wishes about how his affairs should be handled. Precious time together was, by necessity, task oriented instead of meaningful. Had Neil known months before that his timeline was changing, he would have used his final months differently.

Consequences. When patients are not aware of being in the late phase of their illness, the experience turns into what feels like a sudden death, even though it should have been expected. But patients often ignore the signs of decline and miss opportunities to spend their time more beneficially. They are left with anger and regret. They often feel lied to by their health care team and robbed of precious time they would have used differently. Their last chapter of life becomes more a chaotic crisis than a time filled with peace and possibly acceptance. These patients have a sense of unfinished business and no time for proper goodbyes. They may miss the opportunity for life closure. Survivors feel unprepared, shocked, and disbelieving, their grief marked with heightened emotions and decreased coping abilities.

Muriel's Story: In the Know

Muriel is a widow who lived independently at home until she was ninety-six, when her body started to slow down: Her knees were becoming stiffer and sorer, and she was finding it harder to prepare her meals. The few stairs leading outside her home were difficult to manage and she had experienced one frightening fall. Her daughters lived outside the city and they worried about her. So Muriel agreed to move into a retirement home. While there, she made new friends. They sat together for meals in the dining room. Muriel preferred to make a simple breakfast for herself in her room, but she made it to the dining room for lunch and dinner with the help of her walker.

Within two years, Muriel needed help with dressing in the morning and undressing for bed at night. By the following year, she made it to the dining room only for lunch, and the rest of the day, she watched TV in her room. Then she had another fall and ended up in the hospital for a few days. Full investigations in hospital did not reveal any reversible cause to her declining state. When she returned to her retirement home, she was moved to a floor with additional nursing support. She continues to live there as I write, having turned 102 years old recently, but she has really slowed down this past year. She doesn't get to the dining room at all. She needs full help with dressing and bathing. She spends most of her day in her reclining chair, sleeping more than she watches TV. She hasn't had an outing from the retirement home in nine months because of weakness and fatigue. Overall, the speed of her decline seems to be moving monthly at this point. This suggests that Muriel is gently dying and she likely has only months to live. She will continue to slow down, spend more time in bed, eat less, and sleep more. In her final days, she will sleep, sleep, and sleep... and then pass away. This is how most frail elderly people die.

Benefits. When patients have a better sense of their timeline, they have more control in planning for the final chapter of their life. When they understand this transition from the late stage of life to the final chapter, which is the end of life, they approach it with less fear and panic because they know what to expect. The feeling of crisis can be averted by proactive discussion and planning to avoid future falls.

Muriel's daughters know what their mother wants and values, which is to remain in the retirement home for as long as possible. Their hope can evolve realistically, and they can begin to experience anticipatory grief, which prepares them for the future loss of their mother and can have other protective benefits for them.

More broadly, the benefit of knowing that dying has started is that time can be exploited by the patient and family. Time for personal growth, to find meaning and closure, for reconciliation, to grant and receive forgiveness, to say goodbyes. Surprisingly, knowing you have arrived at the late and end stages of an illness can feel both alarming and empowering.

Denial steals away your ability to write your final chapter as you choose. Avoidance robs you of the most precious gift of time—and the ability to decide how you want to use it.

How to Know When Time Is Running Out

No one with a progressive illness can stay hearty indefinitely. Inevitably, the body will slow down. When patients and families don't realize that this is to be expected, it can be extremely frustrating for them. In the more advanced stages of an illness, often the patient and family want to know literally how long they have. They often raise this question when the patient is weighing potentially burdensome treatments, or when they begin to have a gut feeling that their situation is worsening.

It is indeed possible for people to know when they have entered into the late stage of their illness. As mentioned in earlier chapters, each illness has an average prognosis (timeline) based on the millions of people who have already faced the illness. These prognoses, however, are based on population averages and do not necessarily reflect an individual's timeline. An individual's unique timeline is usually not predictable until they are closer to the last year of life. I typically look for the tipping point, when a person starts to show signs of an irreversible decline despite the best underlying medical management of the illness. The more signs I see, the better I can gauge their individual timeline.

Despite differences in each illness, some common features signify when a chronic, progressive illness starts to trend downward. This signals that the patient has entered into the final chapter of life or the advanced stages of the illness. There are three major signals that you've reached the tipping point.

Signal 1: A Decline in Physical Function

A decline in physical function or ability typically involves:

- Weakened physical function. This change can range from being fully able to walk around to reduced mobility, to sitting down most of the time, to mainly lying in bed, to being totally bedbound.
- Increased fatigue or weakness, or decreased stamina.
- Loss of appetite.
- Beginning to have trouble doing basic everyday tasks, also called "activities of daily living" (toileting, bathing, walking, transferring in and out of bed or a chair, eating, and dressing). This can range from doing these tasks independently, to occasionally needing assistance, to requiring considerable assistance, to being totally dependent.
- A need for assistive devices (e.g., wheelchair or walker).

Signal 2: Increase in Patient Needs

This signal may involve:

- Increasing symptoms despite treatment.
- Needing longer appointments.
- Patient requiring help from friend or family member to go to clinic.
- Reaching out to health care team more often for urgent issues.
- Missing appointments because unable or too tired to go to clinic.

Signal 3: Increased Use of Health Care Services

This signal typically involves:

- Unplanned hospital admission(s) or emergency department visits.
- Increased use of oxygen or medical equipment (e.g., a hospital bed).
- Home care and other resources becoming necessary.

Trusting Your Gut

Surprisingly, many patients and families have a gut feeling about approaching end of life. As I mentioned earlier, most patients begin to exhibit a downward decline in the year prior to their death. They express more fatigue, less energy, less appetite. They start to stay home more. They begin to take naps, then more naps. They notice that they don't have the stamina to do what they used to do before. At some point, patients can no longer get to the doctor's office. Many patients describe feeling as though there is a hole in their gas tank and they are running out of gas.

Tip: The speed at which the changes are happening in the last year gently predicts the amount of time a person has left. If you are slowing down from month to month, the prognosis is likely measured in months. If it is changing from week to week, the timeline is likely measured in weeks. If the decline is happening from day to day consistently, then the prognosis is measured in days. Of course, this is just a general estimation, though it has proved to be a very helpful guide. Note that not every change from baseline signals a tipping point. Some changes, especially sudden ones, can signal an acute issue that is potentially treatable.

Therefore, it is important to stress that you are looking for trends, not just one bad month, week, or day. You will want to step back and look for an underlying pattern of decline to help indicate how much time is left.

Action 1: Know the Tipping Point

In discussing the Zoom Out key, I provided details about three main illness trajectories. Each illness trajectory has its own challenges and telltale signs with respect to understanding the overall trends and tipping point. Here, I provide more details about the tipping point for each of the illness trajectories.

The Tipping Point of Steady Decline

In this trajectory, typical of non-curable cancer, one signal that patients are at a tipping point is that they eat less and less because they aren't hungry. They can no longer force themselves to eat enough to sustain their weight. The loss of appetite isn't the cause of the tipping point; it is the consequence of the body starting to prepare for dying. More time is spent at home. They start to feel weaker. During this time, they begin to need more physical support. First, they need help with their regular duties like banking, groceries, lawn and home maintenance, and house cleaning. They may start using a walking aid or wheelchair when distances are too long and exhausting. They need help getting up flights of stairs. They begin to need more personal care as the fatigue and weakness impair them. Eventually, they spend more time sitting and lying down than they do walking. They take longer and longer naps and eat very little. At some point, they begin to feel more comfortable in bed or in a certain chair. Their personal care needs change. For some time, they might be able to be helped to the bathroom. Later, they might transition to using a commode by the chair or bed. Eventually, all care is provided in bed because the patient is so weak that standing or transferring from bed to chair or commode runs a high risk of falling.

During this decline, each patient adjusts to these changes differently. When the changes come without warning or normalizing, patients and family often meet them with a heightened feeling of alarm. If there is no open conversation about these normal changes associated with this wind-down phase, anxiety percolates. My experience has been that once people understand that these changes are to be expected and that this is usually a gentle process over a period of time, their anxiety is mitigated. They feel more trusting, more in control, more knowledgeable, and, as a result, less fearful. Often, the patient considers how and with whom they want to spend their time. Decisions are made about the benefits or burdens of continuing treatments like chemotherapy. Sometimes chemotherapy will continue for a while longer; sometimes it is stopped. It depends on the goal of the treatment and how burdensome it is for the person to continue receiving it. Further appointments for scans and tests are reconsidered because if the story can't be changed, then medical follow-ups aren't a priority anymore. Each situation is different.

When decisions are made to stop treating the underlying illness (e.g., stopping chemotherapy) families and patients might feel as if they've been set adrift. Even so, as the patient continues to decline, families often request scans to reveal the progress of the disease. Truthfully, scans are a less helpful barometer for these purposes than what the family sees right in front of them: the patient's body. For example, a CT scan might conclude that the cancer hasn't grown, but the patient is clearly declining. Alternatively, the CT scan might conclude that the cancer has grown and spread, yet the person is still not showing signs of deterioration. In the final year, evidence of the patient's body succumbing to the illness and its rate of deterioration, not just tests and scans, are the most telling signs of what to expect.

Patients on this illness trajectory generally run a predictable course in the last year. Of all three illness trajectories, this one is the most recognizable in identifying a patient's last year because the decline is more linear.

The Tipping Point of Long Decline with Intermittent Episodes

In this trajectory, the tipping point begins when the symptom exacerbations become worse or more frequent. The trajectory described here, typical of major organ failure, can sometimes be confusing because of the many exacerbations that distract from the background trend downward. With each exacerbation episode, the person doesn't bounce back to their baseline stamina. Just like the cancer trajectory, the decline can be seen in the form of fatigue, weakness, and loss of function. The rate of this overall downward trend is, again, predictive of a timeline. If the decline is happening yearly, monthly, weekly, or daily, the prognosis is, accordingly, yearly, monthly, weekly, or daily. To acknowledge this decline gives those involved important opportunities for conversation about the realities of the illness. Then the focus of care can shift according to the patient's needs and wishes.

The chaos associated with acute exacerbations can be mitigated with thoughtful proactive planning. Each time you have an exacerbation, try to identify the early signs that indicated you were in trouble. What was the treatment plan that got you through the previous episode? This information can be used to predict in a timely fashion when you are headed for trouble. At that time, you can kickstart your action plan to thwart another hospitalization and lessen the burden of each episode. With awareness of the downward trend and exacerbations, improving your quality of life is possible.

So even though patients with end organ failure have an illness pattern marked by severe dips, there is the opportunity to step back and learn from the last exacerbation. The overall trend will still be downward, as with the cancer story, but the exacerbations can be eased. Time spent out of the hospital, at home, with fewer symptoms eases everyone's anxiety and improves quality of life.

Maximizing symptom management and anticipating and planning for acute exacerbations is important throughout this illness trajectory. Again, most patients I meet who are dying of end organ failure die gently. They *can* have a more comfortable course with proper planning and open conversation. Failing this, they often go from one crisis or hospitalization after another.

The Tipping Point of Prolonged Dwindling

In this trajectory, typical of dementia or frailty, the tipping point is much harder to pinpoint because there is an extremely gradual functional decline that occurs over many years. The last year of life for patients dying of frailty and old age is a functional decline much the same as what occurs with each of the other illnesses. Their physical function declines slowly. They require more and more help with activities of daily living, such as bathing, dressing, and feeding. They may even reach a point of near total dependency. As with the other trajectories, the rate of decline predicts the prognosis. Lack of food intake and fatigue are major signs that the person's energy level is declining, and time is running out.

Dementia is one of the main illnesses that follows the trajectory of gradual decline. The average life expectancy for someone diagnosed with dementia is ten years. The inability to coordinate eating, chewing, and swallowing is a hallmark of advanced end-stage dementia. It is often the telltale sign that the patient has entered their last months of life. As with the other illnesses described, patients and families who understand the natural history of the illness' progression are better prepared to deal with the changes when they occur.

Action 2: Update Your Concepts about Palliative Care

It's time to introduce the "P"-word: "palliative care." I know the word "palliative" itself is deeply stigmatized and carries frightening meaning and symbolism for most people. People usually associate palliative care with the end of life. Or the "D"-words, which are "dying" and "death." The mere mention of the word "palliative" usually signals that death is around the corner. This is because, for decades, palliative care was reserved until late in the illness, "when nothing else could be done." No one dared mention it until they were sure they had exhausted all options. At a late point, a person with an advancing illness would suddenly be labeled "palliative" and transferred to a specialist team to receive expert terminal care.

This old-fashioned terminal care model was problematic in many ways. Labeling a patient "palliative" at a late point in time felt like a slap in the face to the patient and family. It felt like a new, deadly diagnosis. Waiting until the end to provide palliative care usually resulted in chaotic crisis care because patients and families had been too long in the dark about the realities of the patient's illness. A sense of hopelessness and abandonment prevailed in this "terminal care" model of delivering palliative care. The other challenge of this model was that it reinforced the outdated notion that nurses and doctors need not have palliative care skills and should transfer the care to someone else—a palliative care specialist—after they determined a "diagnosis" of "palliative."

New Concept

The new concept of palliative care is that it is an *approach* to or a philosophy of care. As defined by the World Health Organization, palliative care "improves the quality of life of patients and their families facing the problems associated with life-threatening illness, through the prevention and relief of suffering by means of early identification and impeccable assessment and treatment of pain and other problems, physical, psychosocial and spiritual." As such, palliative care should not be reserved for the end when all other therapies stop—it is applicable early in the illness, in conjunction with other types of care that are intended to prolong life. Thus, the palliative approach should be incorporated into the entire journey from the beginning, when the patient receives the diagnosis of a life-limiting, progressive illness. Palliative care may be limited at the beginning and increase over time as needed.

Many people assume that palliative care services can be delivered only by palliative care specialists. But palliative care is an approach that should be taught to all nurses and doctors so they know how to seamlessly deliver person-centered care without ever labeling someone "palliative" right before they die. Most agree that the ability to provide the basics of a palliative care approach should be a mandatory skill for all clinicians. In addition, palliative care specialists can be consulted at any point along the journey when complex issues arise.

Since it is a philosophy of care, palliative care is not a diagnosis or a label. People are not "palliative"; patients do not become "palliative."

Research has shown that palliative care is overly associated with patients with cancer diagnoses. Patients with other progressive illnesses, such as advancing heart, lung, neurologic, autoimmune, and kidney diseases, often go unidentified as deserving basic palliative care. So you might have to advocate harder for a palliative approach to care and be more persistent if you have a non-cancer diagnosis.

Tip: Here is a question you can pose to a clinician to trigger a palliative approach to care: "Would you be surprised if I died in the next year?" A family member could also ask this about you. Research shows that when clinicians ask themselves this question, the answer can be remarkably helpful in signaling when a patient is in their last year of life. If the clinician would not be surprised if the patient died within a year, and the patient has exhibited an overall decline with underlying advancing illness, then the patient has likely entered the final chapter of their illness.

Action 3: Try to Appreciate the Silver Lining

There are differences between a sudden and an expected death. When death happens suddenly, perhaps from an accident, there is no opportunity for a life review, purposeful legacy leaving, or saying goodbye or I love you or thank you. Family, neighbors, and coworkers reel in a state of shock. Grieving starts instantly with no time to plan or prepare, and no opportunity to share feelings with the deceased. Many are left with guilt: if they had known it would be the last time they saw the person, they would have said or done something differently or sought forgiveness. They are saddened by the things left unsaid.

In contrast, people who know they are going to die in the near future have an opportunity to plan the time they have left. This goes beyond the concept of checking off items on a bucket list. There is potential to prepare for life closure, a chance to share thoughts with others, settle affairs, and attend to relationships. Some seek to resolve life regrets, connect with estranged family and friends, and take time with friends and relatives to share memories and the importance of their relationships. Many use this time to ensure their family will be cared for after they pass. Importantly, it's an opportunity for family, including young children and friends, to adjust to the reality that their loved one will be gone.

When dying isn't sudden, anticipatory grief usually begins months before, in anticipation of the loss of the loved one. When people see the loss coming, they naturally begin to prepare themselves. It is often an unintentional yet naturally protective coping mechanism. They begin to feel and process the emotions of the impending death. Anticipatory grief doesn't shorten the grieving process but perhaps softens it and allows bereavement to be less complicated for survivors. And because they started grieving before the loss, the bereaved are often better able to move forward after the death compared with those who are mourning a sudden death.

Time is the silver lining of being in the know. Time is precious: it offers opportunity. There's time to be together and to celebrate your life. There's time to decide how you want to spend the next months or weeks. There's time to decide if you want to take that experimental treatment or just be together as a family. There's time to pass on important messages. Many patients write letters to their loved ones for future important dates, like weddings and birthdays. There's time to find meaning, closure, and peace.

Most people dread losing a loved one or being the person who's in their last months or weeks of life. But I can't tell you how many beautiful moments of joy and love I've witnessed during this time. And people wouldn't trade this time for anything. Many patients have told me that in a way, their illness was a gift, that they would never have known otherwise how much someone respected them, or that they meant so much to a person. So again, there is a need to prepare for the last year, and a need for knowledge. If you know what's coming, you can choose however you want to spend the time you have left.

Tip: During this late phase of your illness, you typically need to rely more heavily on your inner crew. The transition from the middle to late phase may be a scary time for you and a scary transition for your inner crew. This is an important time to check in with your inner crew about all the keys in this book, such as what their roles might be moving forward and how they are coping.

Christa's Story: Knowing When Time Was Running Out

I want to share a story from my friend Christa. Her brother-in-law, David, was diagnosed with an aggressive cancer. When she had last seen him, he was very weak. He was unable to walk down the hall without having to stop to catch his breath. People had to hold him up as he was walking. Christa thought death was near and wondered if this was the time when she needed to let the extended family and friends know to say goodbye. But Christa's mother-in-law (David's mother), a nurse for many years who typically spoke openly about death and had been surrounded by it at work her whole life, wasn't saying that the end was near. So Christa second-guessed herself. She emailed me to try to understand what the end of life looked like and what to expect in the final days, since she thought David was at that point but wasn't sure.

I responded with the information in this chapter. She told me, "As soon as I read your email, I knew we didn't have much time left. And I was able to bring my daughter in to see him for the last time. I was confident that I wasn't overreacting in that moment."

When Christa and I spoke months after David died, I asked if, in hindsight, there was evidence that he was beginning to struggle and had approached the tipping point into the late stage of his illness. She pointed out a few clear signs. For example, he had two dogs he adored, and when his parents went to see him, they discovered the dogs had not been walked enough; David couldn't get out of the house regularly to walk them. He also could not handle both dogs being around him at the same time—together, they were too boisterous and energetic for him. Christa said, "When I went to visit his apartment, the way it looked when I got there indicated that things were not well—that he wasn't able to take care of himself and his two pets."

Christa was tuning in to the changing nature of David's condition and readying herself for the inevitable even before she emailed me to ask what the last days of life look like. She told me that David was close to her daughter, his niece. About six weeks before his death, the whole family took a trip to the Dominican Republic with him. In Christa's mind, it was clearly a final family holiday, but no one else talked about it that way. David managed very well on the vacation. He could walk on his own. He had lots of time with Christa's daughter, reading books with her and spending time on the beach. Christa believes David also understood how dire his situation was, and that's why he agreed to go on the trip.

Clearly, coming to terms with the loss of a son or brother is a difficult thing. However, not acknowledging the final chapter can result in different outcomes. Christa admitted that for her husband, David's brother, the death "really took him by surprise." The family was in denial. So when David died, the other family members "did not see it coming." It felt sudden.

I asked if things might have been different at the end if the rest of the family had been more in the know. Christa said yes and gave a few examples. For one, she said, "all of the paperwork for power of attorney and for his will were beside his bed, unsigned, when he died. [The family] knew that they had to do it, but they kept thinking they had more time." Another example was her mother-in-law's guilt about how David's pain was managed at the end. Christa said her mother-in-law "would have administered more pain medication had she known that he was that close to the end. There really wasn't any opportunity for meaningful conversation. She has real regret about that. She worries that he was in so much pain and he could have been more comfortable if they had realized that we were talking days or hours versus weeks and months."

This story is not intended to lay blame on anyone. Dying is difficult. But it is made more difficult when we avoid talking about the inevitable and picking up on the signs in the last year of life. This robs us of time to prepare for the end during the dying process.

When Time Is Running Out: Summary

- Most of us will not die suddenly. Each illness has typical signs that indicate when time is running out. The common sign is when patients begin to exhibit a downward decline without returning to their previous baseline heartiness.
- Palliative care is an approach that focuses on the holistic needs of people; it can start at diagnosis and continue to the end of life. It can be integrated throughout the entire illness trajectory and isn't delivered only by palliative care specialists.
- Recognizing when the end of life is nearing can help bring peace, meaning, and acceptance.

11

DEMYSTIFYING DYING

"By encountering death many thousands of times, I have come to a view that there is usually little to fear and much to prepare for."

KATHRYN MANNIX

THE FINAL PHASE before death, often referred to as the end-of-life or terminal phase, has predictable features regardless of the underlying progressive illness. This chapter debunks misconceptions about the very last weeks and days.

Assumption: Dying Is Agonizing

There is such mystery surrounding dying and death, which comes once in a lifetime for each of us. The world around us shapes our perception and expectations of this mysterious destiny. We get ideas from what we've witnessed by proxy through people dying in our lives or from the media. Television and movies glorify dying and death for more dramatic storytelling, which leaves many people with ill-conceived ideas about dying and death. They think dying is scary, violent, agonizing, and painful.

Reality: Dying Can Be Peaceful

The truth is that most natural dying can be very peaceful.

In the final days and hours, it is normal for families to sit vigil by the bedside, watching their loved one lie peacefully as closely as a new mother watches over her newborn baby as they sleep. It is the time to reconcile that the patient is fading quickly and will soon be gone. This is precious time. In these final moments, families don't need to be burdened by the unknown, fear, and panic.

Dr. Kathryn Mannix, palliative care physician in the UK and bestselling author, writes:

> The death rate remains 100 per cent, and the pattern of the final days, and the way we actually die, are unchanged. What is different is that we have lost the familiarity we once had with that process, and we have lost the vocabulary and etiquette that served us so well in past times, when death was acknowledged to be inevitable. Instead of dying in a dear and familiar room with people we love around us, we now die in ambulances and emergency rooms and intensive care units, our loved ones separated from us by the machinery of life preservation.

Brad and Priya's Story: What Dying Typically Looks Like

Let me explain what the typical end-of-life phase looks like; what a natural death looks like. Brad, a young husband and father of two, was diagnosed with gastric cancer. Specialists treated him with two rounds of chemotherapy over the course of two years. At his last appointment with his oncologist, Brad and his wife, Priya, decided to stop treatment because the cancer was advancing. No other options were available to him. He was gently told, "There is nothing more we can do for you." He was sent home with the subtle message that he would die. Soon after, I was asked to see Brad for the first time because he was experiencing terrible nausea.

Each home is different and the outside and inside offer clues about the patient and how the family is faring. I remember walking up to Brad and Priya's modest semi-detached brick house. It was a sunny spring day. The air was fragrant with lilac trees in full bloom, but the flowers in the pots flanking their front door were long wilted. The garden was overgrown with weeds.

Once inside, I noticed the living room had been reorganized to accommodate Brad's new reclining chair. The couches were pushed aside. The dining room had become a de facto medical supply room. The dining table was covered in cardboard boxes filled with medical supplies. An IV pole stood attached to Brad with a bag of fluid hanging at half-mast. Brad was in pajamas even though it was late afternoon. Priya was in pajamas, too. They apologized for their appearance—they'd had a late start to the day. Brad was finding it difficult to sleep at night, so he slept during the day, they explained. I had a hunch about why he was finding it hard to sleep. The nights were quiet, dark, and lonely. It was probably hard for Brad to keep his mind from worrying then, compared to during the day, with its welcome distractions and the comfort of knowing his family would guard him.

Brad was resting in his reclining chair. He tucked a plastic bowl under his chin in case he vomited. His eyes were large and fearful. He was very thin. Clearly, his weight loss was not new, and I suspected this had started months ago. As I glanced at the family photo on the table beside him, I saw a handsome man beaming at the camera with his wife and children around him. Now, Priya sat on the couch next to him. She was tense.

I am used to people greeting my arrival with caution since I am seen as a harbinger of death. So I pulled up a seat close to Brad. A mentor had taught me to sit no matter how cluttered or impossible it seems in a patient's home. Sitting is calming to everyone and offers a commitment to be truly present.

After a thorough interview and assessment, I was certain that Brad's nausea had both physical and emotional components. He had no appetite at all, but he shared with me that his family encouraged him to eat as much as possible to combat the increasing weakness he'd been feeling over the past couple of months. He was eating "just to put gas in his car, not to satisfy hunger." He admitted that this caused his family a significant amount of distress because they believed "if he didn't eat, he would starve to death." He felt he was letting his family down. Even so, just the smell or mention of food nauseated him. His wife asked me about a feeding tube. "If he can't eat, there has to be a way to get nutrition into him or he'll starve," she insisted.

I knew what they needed. This wasn't about eating; this was about dying. Brad and Priya knew something was happening. They'd noticed changes months earlier but hadn't talked about it for fear of being negative or worrying each other further. Brad and his family had no idea about what to expect during this phase of his illness. They had been discharged from the oncology service with the implied message that he would die at some point, but they had not been told how this part was going to unfold. There is information available to prepare people for the final hours or terminal phase of an illness. However, nothing exists that addresses dying from the time it starts, often a year before a person dies.

I knew what Brad and Priya were wondering. "Will death be painful? Will he suffocate? Will he choke? Will he bleed? Will something shut down?" Patients scan their bodies looking for a sign, the ball to drop, a sudden event. They assume the worst because no one has had an open conversation with them about what to expect. Brad and Priya didn't understand the dying process, so as Brad changed, they interpreted these changes as crises. To them, it was wrong that he had lost his appetite and couldn't eat. And this added to their suffering.

When Brad and Priya were more comfortable in my presence, I asked if they had ever asked their doctors or nurses about what was going to happen next. They lowered their heads and said that they hadn't. I asked them if the doctors or nurses had explained to them what to expect. They said they hadn't. I asked them if they ever wondered about the future and what was going to happen. They both began to weep. I didn't speak; I let them cry for a while. They needed this opportunity for release. I asked them if it would be helpful if I offered some detail about what this phase was going to look like. They looked at each other; both nodded. Priya moved closer to Brad and held his hand with a gentle squeeze. Her other hand held a tissue box. They readied themselves for what they thought I was about to share.

I told Brad that his loss of appetite months before was a common and normal side effect of having cancer. Earlier, he may have been able to continue to encourage himself to eat, but usually this didn't result in weight or energy gain. I shared with him and Priya that forcing him to eat would be futile and only exacerbate his nausea and sense of failure. I explained to Brad that his body had begun the natural process of slowing down. It knew what it was doing. It knew what it needed and didn't need. All the nutrition in the world would not change this process. I paused. This was normal, I explained. I looked at Priya and gently told her that lovingly encouraging Brad to eat would not provide him comfort; in fact, it would contribute to more symptoms and possibly conflict between the two of them. I gave Brad permission to listen to his body, to eat only what he wanted, when he wanted, and the amount he wanted. He said, "Thank you," and looked at Priya to see if she understood. They held each other and cried for a moment.

There was more to tell. I then asked them if they wanted to know more about what to expect. As I anticipated, they nodded. I explained that Brad would continue to feel tired and weak, that this was a usual part of this phase. I told him that he would eat less and drink less and eventually stop doing both. He would sleep more and more. I explained that his body was slowing down. I assured him that dying was usually a gentle process that was preceded by a decline rather than happening in a snap. I explained how the rate of changes in months, weeks, or days usually predicted the time left. At this point, Brad admitted that he was noticing weekly changes.

Priya asked me how to tell when the final days were arriving. I explained that with less food and fluid, Brad would urinate less. In the final forty-eight to seventy-two hours before his passing, his urine might become darker in color because it would be more concentrated. Sometimes this was associated with a stronger smell. Brad would continue to have bowel movements, but these would usually be small and less frequent.

Another sign of the end was that his feet and hands could become cool to the touch because the blood circulation was changing. Brad's skin might also begin to have a purplish patchy look called mottling. Mottling could also occur in the area of the knees, buttocks, and backside. This was normal and not uncomfortable, I assured them.

As his internal chemistry changed, Brad's breathing could take on unique patterns in the final days and hours. It could be fast and shallow, slow and deep, or alternate between both. I explained that it was common for patients to have long pauses in breathing lasting between five and thirty seconds (which for family watching can feel like minutes) before breathing resumed. At this point, patients are asleep and unaware of their breathing patterns. These episodes are called periods of apnea, a telltale sign that death is imminent. I reminded Priya to not shake or nudge Brad to start him breathing again. This would not be effective.

Brad might furrow his brows or open and close his mouth. He might become slightly more restless as death drew closer. This was not pain. It was normal. Sometimes patients seem more confused or fussy in the bed, gesturing with their hands or pulling on their bedclothes. It isn't uncommon for patients to intermittently groan or moan; again, this isn't typically related to pain. This is also normal. I told Priya that during the final stage, Brad's mouth could become very dry, so I told her how to provide mouth care.

I also explained another feature that some families find alarming: wet breathing that might be heard in the final days. Wet breathing doesn't always happen, but when it does, families worry that the lungs are filling up with fluid and that their loved one is drowning or suffocating. This isn't the case. The wet breathing is a result of the natural secretions and saliva that sit at the back of the throat. When a patient is dying, they are too weak to swallow the way healthy people do automatically when their saliva pools. So it just sits there. When the patient is breathing past this saliva, it sounds like gurgling. The sound often worries the family but the breathing is not uncomfortable for the patient. I told Priya that she should not be alarmed if this happens.

I explained that eventually, Brad would take his final breath and slip away.

Brad said, "Are you telling me that eventually I will most likely just fade into a sleep?" I replied yes. He cried with relief. He had assumed that he would die in agonizing pain even though pain had not been part of his experience thus far. Brad and Priya hugged me. They told me I was the first person to speak to them so honestly.

I spent over an hour in Brad and Priya's home. During that time, we talked about his symptoms. We reviewed his many medications, including three prescribed for his nausea, which we stopped because his nausea would end when he no longer forced himself to eat. But for most of the visit, we discussed his illness from beginning to end. We put together the pieces of information to map out his journey. We discussed the current stage of his illness (advanced) and what to expect—the changes they would notice that are a normal part of this journey. We discussed his timeline, not just based on statistics, but on his individual presentation. We discussed what would be available to them for assistance as Brad's situation changed. We discussed the children and how to communicate with them. We put action plans in place in anticipation of foreseeable issues. I told them whom to call whenever they had a concern. Essentially, we openly discussed what dying looks like.

Brad and Priya were appreciative and relieved. They felt calmer, even though they were grieving. Their fears and anxieties were diminished considerably just because they had been gently invited into a conversation about something they had been wondering about for months.

They were visibly more at ease when their kids arrived home from school. Brad died less than two weeks later, comfortably at home. His nausea had disappeared without additional prescribed medications. It had been treated with conversation.

Common Misconceptions about Dying

There are many other common misconceptions about dying. They always stem from a fundamental gap in real information. The chasm between truth and falsehood starts when we are young and builds momentum over our lives. These myths have a cumulative effect—from the time of a serious diagnosis to the end—and complicate the illness journey. Seeking factual information about what to expect is the best insurance for retaining your sense of self, staying in control, and feeling dignified until the end.

Much of my work is spent demystifying dying for health care providers, patients, and families. Failure to address the myths, misconceptions, and misinformation that cloud the topic of dying and death results in misguided decision-making, decreased quality of life, and increased suffering.

In the rest of the chapter, I will tackle other common misconceptions about dying and death.

Myth: Talking about Dying Causes Hopelessness

There is a strongly held belief that people will automatically lose all hope if they know they are dying, that they'll give up the fight. This is not necessarily true but is more likely to be the case if we fool people into believing they will beat the illness. On one hand, the longer it takes to have open conversations about the reality of the illness, the more potential there is for hopelessness when the truth is obvious. On the other hand, people who are guided along with knowledge about what is happening to them can shift their hope as their situation changes. Patients who are stuck in unrealistic hope become hopeless because the focus of hope doesn't evolve with the reality of the illness.

It has been my experience that when talking with patients about the gravity of their illness, it's important to assess their individual need and readiness for information about the gentle truth. If they are spoken with proactively, with honesty and kindness, patients and families usually feel more empowered with accurate information about their current and future state. This is true even if the information isn't "good news." You may need time to adjust, but eventually you will feel relieved that people are speaking more honestly about your situation.

With respect to depression, studies estimate that the prevalence of clinical depression for people with advanced illness is approximately 30 percent. That means that 70 percent of people don't develop clinical depression even though they are facing a progressive illness. This doesn't mean people don't feel sad, worried, anxious, frustrated, or scared at times throughout their illness; but most don't slip into a depression. Remarkably, most people maintain a sense of hope, worth, and meaning throughout their journey. Most can find some reason their life is still worth living right until the end, regardless of how simple and small their pleasures might be.

So, it *isn't* true that when a person has a progressive, life-limiting illness, they will naturally and understandably be depressed. The assumption that depression is a normal part of dying can lead to a problem for those patients who do truly suffer from depression. If it is considered normal, then we may not take it seriously, and as a result, patients with true depression may not access the proper supports. It is important to address depression seriously when it *is* present and not assume it to be just part of the journey. But at the same time, it's striking that roughly 70 percent of patients facing progressive illness don't get depressed!

Myth: Dying Is Painful

Most people assume that dying is automatically painful. But this is not necessarily true. The underlying physiologic process of dying itself, when the body naturally slows down, is not painful. But you do have to consider what the illness is. Each illness has a different potential for pain along the journey. And every person has a unique pain threshold. Two people with the same illness can have completely different pain experiences.

You should also consider how you have fared with this illness so far. A person's past pattern of symptoms usually signals the types of challenges they will face when dying. For example, if your pain has been hard to control, it may continue to be a challenge. Fortunately, medications can often lessen the severity of symptoms so they aren't impeding a patient's ability to have a good quality of life. Alternatively, if you have had very little pain, you are unlikely to have worse pain when you are winding down.

Even if pain is a potential hurdle, careful planning for anticipated pain can downgrade a perceived crisis into a manageable event. Proactively creating a pain plan that is tailored to the ability of your first responder, often an untrained family member, is helpful in averting a pain crisis. Caregivers need to know about expected issues and what to do in what-if scenarios—for example, how to administer breakthrough or rescue pain medications or how to get and use the symptom relief kit for the home. The bottom line is: unbearable pain is not a given near death.

Further, there is a related myth that taking pain medications can lead to addiction or hasten death. The main goal at end of life is the patient's comfort and managing if there is pain related to the advancing disease. Clinicians have expertise to use the right drugs, in the right way, and in the right doses so they are safe and effective. Using pain medications, such as morphine, will not hasten death when used properly. Patients are dying because of their disease, not because of the pain medications. The medications are given to address pain and other symptoms, so the patient is more comfortable.

Again, dying itself is not painful. It can be very comfortable because of the absence of pain altogether or the management of pain.

Myth: Symptoms Will Automatically Worsen as Death Nears

Symptoms typically don't escalate during this declining phase. Depending on the underlying illness, people can experience a variety of symptoms throughout their illness. Symptoms may be directly caused by the illness itself (like breathlessness from heart failure), by the treatment for the illness (like nausea from chemotherapy), or by the person's changing condition (like fatigue). However, I have met many people who have very little symptom burden throughout their entire journey. The decline while dying is not always accompanied by symptoms. The most common symptoms are fatigue and weakness.

The pattern of the patient's previous symptoms, whether shortness of breath, nausea, or something else, usually foretells how symptomatic the person will be throughout the rest of the illness. Symptoms don't usually appear just because a person is deteriorating. So if the symptoms have been mild all along, they usually remain mild throughout the illness.

As well, my experience has been that symptoms are not necessarily correlated to the patient's scans. Sometimes scans look awful, but the patient has few symptoms. Other times, the scans look stable, yet the patient is having more symptoms.

I've also come to appreciate that symptoms can be significantly amplified by emotions, fears, and worries. Patients and families seem to be more comfortable expressing physical symptoms than talking about their feelings. It is widely accepted that there is a strong link between the mind and body. Part of treating physical symptoms is making sure that other stressors and emotions are attended to.

If new or worsening symptoms do occur, proper assessment is paramount because many causes of symptoms can be treated. Symptoms are multifactorial, so if they seem to be escalating unexpectedly, I always assess for underlying psychosocial factors.

I can't say that it is always smooth going. But most of the challenges that potentially make this part of the journey rocky are peripheral to dying. For example, issues related to a lack of clinician assessment skills, a lack of clinician knowledge in providing care in this phase, inappropriate treatment options in the absence of a full discussion about the big picture, fewer optimal choices of symptom management treatments, inappropriate doses of medications, miscommunication, and fear and panic are more likely to make the last year rocky. Most people rush to the emergency department because they don't understand what's happening.

Possible hurdles, such as sudden problems, that disrupt a gentle decline can often be predicted by simply looking at the patient's journey thus far. If a patient has had episodes of vomiting, then it can be anticipated that this might happen again, but not necessarily. If a patient has had multiple chest infections, then this might happen again, but not necessarily. Looking retrospectively for trends can help plan for future potential issues and guide preparation.

Myth: Patients Who Stop Eating Are Starving to Death

The role of nutrition throughout an illness changes. In the beginning, ensuring that a patient receives enough calories to sustain their weight helps them hold up to treatments, recover from surgery, maintain energy and healing, and prevent or repair wounds. As the illness progresses to the more advanced stages, patients often lose their appetite and consequently eat less and less. When the body is dying, it is programmed to know how to wind down.

I would estimate that in my own practice, families raise questions related to nutrition and hydration in at least three-quarters of my visits. Weight loss is often a harbinger of dying and can cause a significant amount of distress and conflict between patients and families. It is very important that patients and families understand the underlying cause of low appetite and weight loss because it usually coincides with the patient beginning to wind down. This is not starving to death or giving up; this is dying.

If not told otherwise, patients and families think the loss of appetite causes the patient's deterioration. But the wind-down, low energy, fatigue, and low appetite are symptoms, not causes of, the changes happening internally because of the underlying disease. Often, once the appetite dips, the changes are irreversible. Additional food does not fix the problem, which is not lack of nutrition.

As Brad's example showed, a person who is actively dying does not eat or drink. Additional intake of calories in the final months does not improve energy, fatigue, or weight gain. In fact, when active dying begins and until the end, encouraging food and fluid can be uncomfortable, even counterproductive, for a person who has no appetite. Some family members struggle with this concept so much so that they try to force the person to eat or drink, despite that the patient is too sleepy and too weak to swallow. The food could potentially be misdirected into the lungs instead of the stomach and this can cause pneumonia.

Too much fluid can cause uncomfortable swelling of the legs and complicate caregiving (heavy turning and repositioning).

Low appetite and weight loss can also be very disturbing for patients. Patients might feel like they aren't trying hard enough, thus failing their loved ones and clinicians. Many are embarrassed about how they look and begin to stay home more. Some miss the social aspects of eating with others and even simply miss the routine of eating. If the patient is overly distressed by this, medications can be used to try to stimulate or trick a person's body into feeling a sense of appetite. However, in the advanced stages, this will *not* change the course of decline. Patients, on average, don't usually live longer than seven to ten days without any fluid. This timeline helps families with their planning.

Myth: "Do Not Resuscitate" Means Giving Up All Treatment

People believe that opting out of CPR, such as signing a Do Not Resuscitate (DNR) form, means no longer receiving any care. Relatedly, many assume that choosing "no heroic measures" means that any and all treatments are being abandoned. However, heroic measures are limited to few specific interventions, such as having a feeding tube, intubation, CPR, or a ventilator.

The reality is that even in the absence of resuscitation or other heroic measures, you can still get attentive care. Be assured that a DNR form doesn't mean that health care professionals are giving up on you. Instead, by signing a DNR, you are specifically indicating that should your heart stop for any reason, you do not want health care professionals to attempt resuscitation.

Despite what you might see in a Hollywood movie, resuscitation in the context of advanced terminal illness does *not* result in the person pulling through and returning to their baseline. When a person begins to decline in the final year of life, resuscitation is highly unlikely to be successful. It does not prevent the inevitable. At best, a person might end up on life-support machines; they will never live with the quality of life they had previously. This is why I encourage my patients and families to understand the incredibly low odds of a successful resuscitation; in a crisis, some people tend to choose resuscitation out of fear that they won't receive any other care to keep them comfortable.

The alternative to a "full code," which includes all means to keep a person alive (for example, CPR) is comfort care measures or Allow Natural Death (AND). Comfort care measures and Allow Natural Death are the same as opting for no heroic measures or life-sustaining interventions. However, they allow active care that is focused on maintaining quality of life and comfort.

Myth: Dying Should Be Hidden from Children

Our instinct is to shield children from harm, so naturally adults tend to protect young ones from the knowledge that a loved one is dying. Just like denial, this results in a short-term solution until, suddenly, the loved one is gone and reality hits the children head-on. After all, you can only hide dying until the person is dead—then there is a lot of explaining to do. Kids are more perceptive than we give them credit for. Many children in the home of loved ones who are declining can see that something is changing and often wonder why the adults are behaving the way they do. Children often wonder, "Why do the grown-ups who have been sad suddenly jump up and smile when I enter the room? Why do I get shooed out every time I'm around? Why is no one talking to me about what is happening?"

I am often asked, "What or when should we tell our children about what's happening?" I usually share with families that the literature on this topic suggests that adults take their cues from the children, and that this needs to be individualized. How dying is communicated to children needs to be done in the context of their age, maturity, and level of interest and curiosity about what is happening. The explanation needs to be tailored to the intellectual ability of the child. Language is important. Fortunately, there are wonderful resources in the children's section of the library that are specifically geared to varying ages. Often, age-appropriate stories of death and dying give children the opportunity to ask questions.

Generally, children fare better during the final months, days, and hours when they are permitted to be around and involved in the event as much as they want. That said, although it is common for some children to want to stay close by, others prefer to be at a distance. Each child is different, but each should be invited to be present if they wish. When children are gently included in the reality of a declining illness, the inevitable death doesn't feel like such a shock and they deal with the immediate death feeling sad but safe among trusted adults. Interestingly, people who were shielded from a death in the family when they were young often share with me that they still feel regret and guilt into their adult lives.

Demystifying Dying: Summary

- Watching the decline before death is alarming unless the patient and family know what is normal and to be expected. The temptation is to "do" and "fix" to prolong the inevitable.
- Knowing what to expect and what dying looks like, although emotionally taxing, puts patients and families in better control. They can plan and coordinate care and choose how they want to spend their time.

- Most people die over a period of time and gently. With careful proactive planning, rarely does a person die with a huge symptom burden. The main features of dying are weakness, fatigue, low appetite, and sleep.

CONCLUSION

NO MATTER what type of life-changing diagnosis you have, using the seven keys early will give you knowledge, which is the best way to maintain control and power over your illness journey. A typical health care journey can leave people feeling scared, broken down, defeated, and unrecognizable. Being in the know is your best insurance for remaining a whole person while in the role of patient.

The other thing the keys give you is the gift of time. Time allows you to prepare. If you know enough early on, time allows you to find the silver lining of having a serious diagnosis. Don't wait for a crisis to practice all seven keys at once. By then, it is often too late to derive the benefit they can offer. You can only control so much, especially with a life-changing diagnosis. But the keys, when used early on, will give you a hidden power of knowledge and preparation that will allow you to truly be activated in your illness experience.

Being an activated and informed patient goes against the grain, which can be difficult. It's revolutionary. That's why this book is part of larger social movement, the Waiting Room

Revolution. By implementing the seven keys early on in your illness, you'll become a trailblazer of sorts. You'll be a new type of patient. Not just by having more knowledge but by contextualizing that knowledge for your own life—the meaning-making behind all the facts.

But it's not going to be easy. Don't be surprised if, when you use the seven keys with your health care providers, you're met with lots of different reactions. The reactions are going to depend on those other people's styles and experiences, how awake they are to the challenges in the system, and how urgent things seem. Be ready for pushback, deflection, and "kick the can down the road" kind of responses. It may not be smooth sailing from the start.

But persist. Because it's important. It's your life.

You Are Not Alone

If you and others heed my advice, and suddenly many patients go forward activated, it will shock the health care system, which is going to take some time to adapt. That doesn't mean you stop.

As far as I can see, this is the only way forward. It is the only way to create large-scale change in a complex health and social system. It is the only way to shift things so every patient and family can change the default experience of being in the dark to a standard of being in the know.

Remember that you are not alone. All around you, patients are going through a similar journey or they have already walked it before you. They are your allies. So, too, are future patients, who are often in the role of caregiver or carer or "family." They are on a related journey.

My final advice: What I've learned from years of educating health care providers is that knowledge without action doesn't lead to change. So take action. Small steps can lead to big change when you keep consistent and remain proactive. Keep inviting yourself to the conversation. When you do, you will get more answers. You will be less in the dark and more in the know. More able to hope for the best and plan for the rest.

ACKNOWLEDGMENTS

MY COAUTHOR, Hsien Seow, and I have many people to thank for helping us bring this dream into reality. First and foremost, we want to thank our families, who have supported us at every step. They are our rocks and our hearts. Sammy wants to thank Mitchell; Lauren; Sarah; her parents, Susan and Mickey; and her "slow walking crew." Hsien wants to thank Katie, Hannah, Miya, Kelvin, Linda, and his parents, Suat Tein and Pau Chern.

This book, which is connected to the Waiting Room Revolution, has been the result of the tireless efforts of the McMaster University research team, including Shilpa Jyothi Kumar, Valerie Bishop, Wanda Oldfield, Daryl Bainbridge, Ana Dos Santos, and Sue Tan Toyofuku. We want to especially thank Maggie Civak and Kayla McMillan, who were instrumental in helping us clarify our ideas for this book.

Thank you to those who supported our writing at various stages: Christa Haanstra, Paul Adams, Paul LaLonde, Sylvia Hagopian, Christina Frangou, Amy Tan, Nick Kates, and Sam Hiyate. We are grateful for the entire publishing team at Page Two, especially Trena White, for believing in us from the start, and her amazing team, including Kendra Ward, Caela Moffet, Meghan O'Neill, Jennifer Lum, and Lorraine Toor.

We are forever indebted to the many patients, families, and health care providers who shared their stories with us for this book, on our podcast, and at the bedside. They offered intimate details about their lives with the goal to help others; we hope we have done them justice.

Lastly, thank you to everyone supporting us in the Waiting Room Revolution social movement—on social media and podcasts, through email, and with conference invites. You helped us turn this dream into a movement.

NOTES

Chapter 1: From "In the Dark" to "In the Know"

p. 21 *But psychology research shows that any information:* A. Tversky and E. Shafir, "The Disjunction Effect in Choice under Uncertainty," *Psychological Science* 3, no. 5 (1992): 305–9, doi.org/10.1111/j.1467-9280.1992.tb00678.x.

Chapter 2: Walk Two Roads

p. 29 *providers and patients don't talk about preparing for the rest:* L. Granek, M.K. Krzyzanowska, R. Tozer, et al., "Oncologists' Strategies and Barriers to Effective Communication about the End of Life," *Journal of Oncology Practice* 9, no. 4 (2013): e129–35, doi.org/10.1200/JOP.2012.000800.

p. 30 *honest conversations about the future reduce anxiety and depression:* J.S. Temel, J.A. Greer, A. Muzikansky, et al., "Early Palliative Care for Patients with Metastatic Non-Small-Cell Lung Cancer," *New England Journal of Medicine* 363, no. 8 (2010): 733–42, doi.org/10.1056/NEJMoa1000678.

p. 30 *toxic positivity is not a healthy way to deal with challenges:* Z. Villines, "What to Know about Toxic Positivity," Medical News Today, March 30, 2021, medicalnewstoday.com/articles/toxic-positivity.

Chapter 3: Zoom Out

p. 59 *each illness has a different rhythm and pattern to it:* J.R. Lunney, J. Lynn, D.J. Foley, et al., "Patterns of Functional Decline at the End of Life," *Journal of the American Medical Association* 289, no. 18 (2003): 2387–92, doi.org/10.1001/jama.289.18.2387.

Chapter 5: Customize Your Order

p. 103 *Some prescriptions or treatments may not be covered by your insurance:* F. Chino, "My Unfortunate Introduction Into the Financial Toxicity of Cancer Care in America—March Forth," *JAMA Oncology* 4, no. 5 (2018): 628–29, doi.org/10.1001/jamaoncol.2017.4436.

p. 111 *ask yourself a modified version of the Patient Dignity Question:* H.M. Chochinov, *Dignity Therapy: Final Words for Final Days* (New York: Oxford University Press, 2011).

Chapter 6: Anticipate Ripple Effects

p. 123 *More than one in four Canadians are currently caregivers:* M. Sinha, *Portrait of Caregivers, 2012*, Spotlight on Canadians: Results from the General Social Survey analytical paper (Ottawa, ON: Statistics Canada, September 2013), www150.statcan.gc.ca/n1/en/pub/89-652-x/89-652-x2013001-eng.pdf?st=qLwUTjjJ.

p. 123 *A 2020 national US survey:* AARP and the National Alliance for Caregiving, *Caregiving in the U.S.: 2020 Report* (Washington, DC: AARP, May 2020), aarp.org/content/dam/aarp/ppi/2020/05/full-report-caregiving-in-the-united-states.doi.10.26419-2Fppi.00103.001.pdf.

p. 124 *approximately 75 to 80 percent of people's care occurs outside a hospital:* R.W. Johnson and J.M. Wiener, *A Profile of Frail Older Americans and Their Caregivers,* The Retirement Project—Occasional Paper No. 8 (Washington, DC: Urban Institute, February 2006), urban.org/sites/default/files/publication/42946/311284-A-Profile-of-Frail-Older-Americans-and-Their-Caregivers.PDF.

Chapter 7: Connect the Dots

p. 161 *This negative experience motivated Karen and her sister to write a book:* K. Cumming and P. Milne, *The Indispensable Survival Guide to Ontario's Long-Term Care System: Practical Tips to Help You and Your Family Be Proactive and Prepared* (Victoria, BC: Tellwell Talent, 2019).

Chapter 8: Invite Yourself

p. 167 *Research suggests that doctors are hesitant to discuss bad news:* W.I. Zhi and T.J. Smith, "Early Integration of Palliative Care into Oncology: Evidence, Challenges and Barriers," *Annals of Palliative Medicine* 4, no. 3 (2015): 122–31, doi.org/10.3978/j.issn.2224-5820.2015.07.03.

p. 171 *implementing what she calls the TEAM approach:* C. Snyman, *Two Steps Forward: Embracing Life with a Brain Tumor* (Vancouver, BC: Two Steps Publishing, 2015).

p. 185 *a vocal caregiving and disability advocate and author:* D. Thomson and Z. White, *The Unexpected Journey of Caring: The Transformation from Loved One to Caregiver* (Lanham, MD: Rowman & Littlefield, 2019).

Chapter 9: Putting It All Together

p. 196 *Gaps in care for racialized and LGBTQ2IA+ communities:* See, for example, R. Casanova-Perez, C. Apodaca, E. Bascom, et al., "Broken Down by Bias: Healthcare Biases Experienced by BIPOC and LGBTQ+ Patients," *AMIA Annual Symposium Proceedings* (2021): 275–284, ncbi.nlm.nih.gov/pmc/articles /PMC8861755/pdf /3576813.pdf.

Chapter 10: When Time Is Running Out

p. 203 *only 10 percent of us will die an unexpected, sudden death:* M. Heron, "Deaths: Leading Causes for 2019," *National Vital Statistics Reports* 70, no. 9 (2021): 1–114, dx.doi.org/10.15620/cdc:107021.

p. 216 *As defined by the World Health Organization, palliative care:* World Health Organization and Worldwide Palliative Care Alliance, *Global Atlas of Palliative Care at the End of Life* (London, UK: Worldwide Hospice Palliative Care Alliance, 2014), iccp-portal.org/system/files /resources/Global_Atlas_of_Palliative_Care.pdf.

p. 217 *palliative care is overly associated with patients with cancer diagnoses:* K.L. Harrison, A.A. Kotwal, and A.K. Smith, "Palliative Care for Patients with Noncancer Illnesses," *Journal of the American Medical Association* 324, no. 14 (2020): 1404–5, doi.org/10.1001/jama.2020.15075.

p. 217 *Research shows that when clinicians ask themselves this question:* R.D. Romo and J. Lynn, "The Utility and Value of the 'Surprise Question' for Patients with Serious Illness," *Canadian Medical Association Journal* 189, no. 33 (2017): e1072–73, doi.org/10.1503/cmaj.733231.

Chapter 11: Demystifying Dying

p. 226 *Dr. Kathryn Mannix, palliative care physician:* K. Mannix, *With the End in Mind: How to Live and Die Well* (Glasgow, UK: William Collins, 2018), 2.

p. 234 *With respect to depression, studies estimate:* A.J. Mitchell, M. Chan, H. Bhatti, et al., "Prevalence of Depression, Anxiety, and Adjustment Disorder in Oncological, Haematological, and Palliative-Care Settings: A Meta-Analysis of 94 Interview-Based Studies," *Lancet Oncology* 12, no. 2 (2011): 160–74, doi.org/10.1016/S1470-2045(11)70002-X.

ABOUT THE AUTHORS

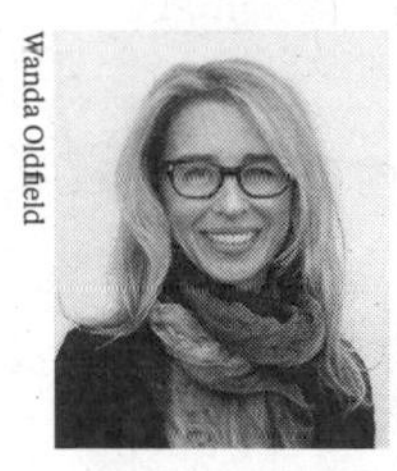

Wanda Oldfield

DR. SAMMY WINEMAKER is a palliative care physician who cares for patients with serious illness and their families in the home. She is an associate clinical professor at McMaster University in the Department of Family Medicine, Division of Palliative Care. She has won numerous awards for her leadership and palliative care education for health care professionals.

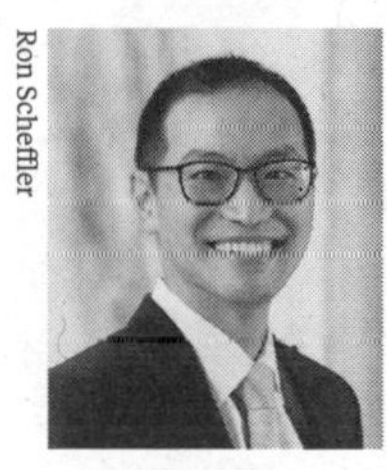

Ron Scheffler

DR. HSIEN SEOW is the Canada Research Chair in Palliative Care and Health System Innovation and a professor in the Department of Oncology at McMaster University. He publishes health care research focused on improving the patient and family experience for those facing serious illness. He is the coauthor of *The Tao of Innovation: Nine Questions Every Innovator Must Answer.*

OUR INVITATION TO YOU

This book is part of a larger social movement called the Waiting Room Revolution. Everyone is invited, including you, to join the movement. The movement is a community where you can learn more and engage with other patients and caregivers.

Four Ways to Join the Waiting Room Revolution

Join our email list: Stay up-to-date on upcoming events, novel patient tools, and new ventures by joining our mailing list at waitingroomrevolution.com.

Listen to *The Waiting Room Revolution* podcast: We interview a diverse group of people from all over the world who share their advice and stories. Rate and review us wherever you get your podcasts.

Share with others: This book was designed to be read with others. Discuss the exercises with family and friends or host a book club. Let us know how it goes.

Invite us: We are happy to speak at conferences, webinars, or other community events or workshops. Send us an email.

Connect with Us

waitingroomrev@gmail.com

waitingroomrevolution.com

@WaitingRoomRev, @SammyWinemaker, @HSeowPhD, #HopeForTheBest

Samantha Winemaker, Hsien Seow

@sammy.winemaker

@WaitingRoomRev

@dr.sammywinemaker

THE GLORIES OF HEAVEN

THE GLORIES OF HEAVEN

The Supernatural Gifts that Await Body & Soul in Paradise

ST. ANSELM *of* CANTERBURY

TRANSLATED BY

FR. ROBERT NIXON, OSB

TAN Books
Gastonia, North Carolina

Translated by Fr. Robert Nixon, OSB

Cover design by www.davidferrisdesign.com

Cover image: Detail of the painting of the interior of the dome depicting the Holy Trinity, 1663-65 / Mignard, Pierre / © Clement Guillaume / Bridgeman Images

ISBN: 978-1-5051-2711-9
Kindle ISBN: 978-1-5051-2712-6
ePUB ISBN: 978-1-5051-2713-3

Published in the United States by
TAN Books
PO Box 269
Gastonia, NC 28053
www.TANBooks.com

Printed in the United States of America

O my Friend, flee for a while from your occupations;
Hide yourself from the tumult of your thoughts.
Cast aside your burdensome cares and put off
your laborious duties.
Rest in God, and take your ease in Him.
Enter the inner chamber of your mind;
Shut out everything except for God, and whatever
helps you to find Him.
Close the door firmly and seek Him.
Say now, my heart, say to God:
"I seek Thy face; Thy face, O Lord, do I seek."

—*Saint Anselm,* Proslogion

CONTENTS

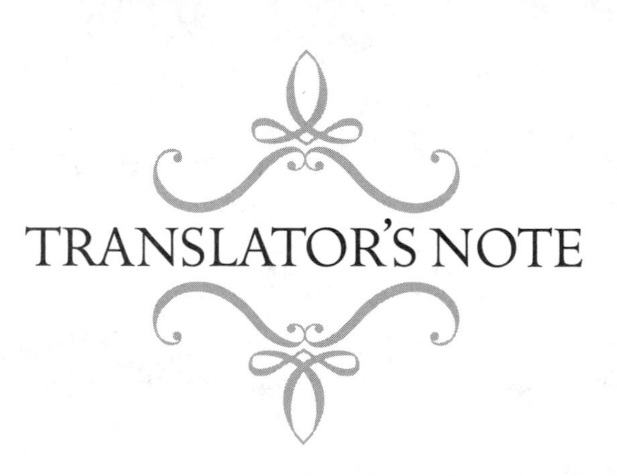

TRANSLATOR'S NOTE

SAINT ANSELM OF Canterbury (1033–1109) occupies a distinguished position amongst the great ecclesiastical leaders and spiritual and theological luminaries who have adorned the Benedictine Order. His *Proslogion* (articulating the famous "ontological argument" for God's existence), *Monologion*, and the treatise *Cur Deus Homo* (*Why God Became Human*) are all indispensable and foundational reading for any serious student of theology. Yet, apart from the learned philosophical and theological works of this illustrious Doctor of the Church, Anselm also produced a very considerable corpus of profound and moving mystical and devotional writings. One such work, which is of particular importance and beauty, is presented in this volume in English translation for the first time: *De Beatitudine Coelestis Patriae* (*On the Beatitude of the Celestial Homeland*, entitled here *The Glories of Heaven: The Supernatural Gifts that Await Body and Soul in Paradise*).

The Glories of Heaven is a transcription of a conference given by Anselm to the monks at the great monastery of Cluny in France. The actual scribe is identified as the monk Eadmer of Canterbury. This Eadmer was a friend and student of Anselm, and he also wrote his most complete and authoritative biography. In the course of this extended conference, Anselm describes systematically various aspects of the happiness of heaven. Although the joys of heaven necessarily transcend and surpass all that can possibly be imagined or expressed, the author postulates that whatever brings us joy during our earthly life will also be present in heaven, but extrapolated there to an infinite degree both in intensity and duration. Thus all the joys experienced in passing and fragmentary form in the here-and-now will be given to us in complete fullness and perfection in the life of eternity.

The spiritual value of the contemplation of the glories of heaven perhaps tends to be overlooked by many contemporary Christians. Yet it is a powerful and potent source of motivation, encouragement, and consolation. Saint Benedict, in his *Rule,* urges us to "yearn for everlasting life with holy desire."[1] Anselm's eloquent conference on this subject certainly serves to enliven such holy desires and to awaken such noble yearnings.

In addition, Anselm's *Mediation on the Day of Judgment and the Blessings of Heaven* and *Exhortation to Strive for the*

---

1 *Rule of St. Benedict*, 4:46.

Glories of Heaven are included here. These works, which continue to treat the theme of the glories and joys of heaven, present a spirituality which is radically eschatological. Namely, Anselm urges the reader to live in a manner which is oriented towards future and eternal realities. We witness in these short treatises Anselm's legendary skills as a homilist. His powerful and resonant words can hardly fail to move the soul to a holy desire for the blessings and peace of paradise and the radiant splendors of the New Jerusalem.

As well as these fascinating and inspiring works, a translation of the biography of Saint Anselm from the Tridentine *Breviarium Romanum* is included in this volume.

Anselm of Canterbury, the "*Doctor Magnificus*," was a saint who united the mysticism and austerity of the contemplative and monastic life with the zeal and pastoral diligence of apostolic and episcopal ministry. His writings similarly unite penetrating intelligence and clear, analytical reasoning with overflowing and ardent devotion and passionate imagination. May they continue to guide today's readers in their search for God and inflame in our hearts a desire for the joys and glories of our celestial homeland. And may Saint Anselm intercede for each of us and for the holy Catholic Church. Amen.

Fr. Robert Nixon, OSB
Abbey of the Most Holy Trinity
New Norcia, Western Australia

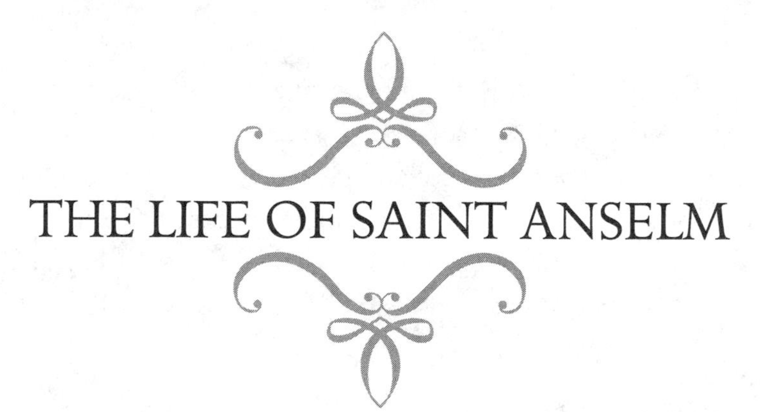

THE LIFE OF SAINT ANSELM

from the Breviarium Romanum: ex decreto SS. Concilii Tridentini restitutum

SAINT ANSELM WAS born to noble parents, Gundulph [his father] and Ermemberg [his mother], in Aosta[1] in Italy. From his tender years, he was infused with a desire for holiness of life as well as an ardent love of literary studies, and even as a child, he gave many clear signs of his future sanctity and learning.

While he was a youth, however, his attentions were diverted by the vain allurements of this passing world, as is so often the case with young people. But this period of distraction lasted only for a short time, and very soon his heart returned to the narrow path of righteousness. Inspired by

[1] A city in the Italian alpine region.

the desire to attain true sanctity, he left his family's riches and high status and entered the monastery of the Order of Saint Benedict at Bec.[2] There he made his monastic vows under the Abbot Heluin. Lanfranc,[3] the most learned man of his time, served as his teacher and mentor at the monastery. Under his wise direction, Anselm applied himself both to his studies and the cultivation of virtue with such zeal that he made miraculous progress. He soon came to be an exemplar both of learning and holiness to the entire monastic community.

He was so assiduous in his practice of fasting that it seemed as if all sense of taste for food had been rendered extinct in him. He occupied himself diligently in his monastic duties, unceasingly either teaching or responding to various questions and uncertainties on matters of religion and theology. During the night, he took additional time from the hours of sleep to apply himself to silent meditation on divine things. By doing this, he constantly refreshed his soul with the life-giving nourishment of prayer, tears, and holy contemplation.

When he was elected prior of the community, he encountered much envy and resentment from certain brothers. Yet his humility, charity, and prudence were so great

---

[2] Located in Normandy in France.

[3] Blessed Lanfranc was regarded as the leading Latinist and theologian of his time, and was a prolific writer.

and unwavering that he soon won the respect and affection of these brothers, and thus turned his former enemies and rivals into his loyal friends. He inspired all the brethren to the deepest love of God and most zealous observance of the monastic rule.

After the death of the abbot of his monastery, Anselm was elected as abbot himself—a position which he accepted with a reluctance born of true humility. Very soon, his reputation for sound doctrine and sanctity spread, and his fame shone forth like a radiant light. Not only kings and bishops held him in veneration and esteem, but even the pope, Saint Gregory VII, wrote to him in letters filled with love and admiration. Now at that time, the Church was suffering from very grave persecutions and much internal turmoil, so the Roman pontiff earnestly entreated Anselm to pray both for him and for the entire Catholic Church.[4]

[Now, Lanfranc, Anselm's former teacher at the monastery at Bec, had been chosen as archbishop of Canterbury some time previously and had served in this role with great distinction.] When Lanfranc passed away, Anselm was urged to take up this position, both by William, the king of England,[5] and all the people and clergy of that land.

---

4 At this time, the Roman Church (and Pope Gregory VII in particular) was in conflict with the Holy Roman emperor, Henry IV, who supported a rival claimant to the papacy, the antipope Clement III.

5 This was probably William I, or William the Conqueror, the Duke of Normandy who had invaded England in 1066.

Anselm was at first unwilling to accept such an elevated ecclesiastical dignity; yet, prompted by so many appeals, he reluctantly agreed.

Immediately, he set to work trying to improve the morals of the general population and also to improve discipline within the Church. This he did both by preaching and by writing, and by convening various councils.

But he came into conflict with King William,[6] who tried to infringe the freedom and rights of the Church by force. With true priestly constancy, Anselm resisted him firmly. As a consequence, churches and monasteries were stripped of many of their assets, and Anselm himself was forced into exile.

So, banished from England, he traveled to Rome, where he was received with great honor by Pope Urban II. He participated actively in the Council of Barens, arguing convincingly, on the basis of innumerable references to Scripture and the writings of the Church Fathers, that the Holy Spirit proceeded from both the Father and the Son. This was to disprove the error of the Greeks [who believed that the Holy Spirit proceeds from the Father alone and not from the Son.]

Once King William [II] had passed away, Anselm was recalled to England by the new monarch, King Henry, who was the brother of the deceased William. Shortly after his

---

[6] This seems to have been Willian II, the son of William the Conqueror.

return to England, Anselm passed away peacefully. His fame spread very quickly—both for miracles and outstanding sanctity. This sanctity included particularly his fervent devotion towards the blessed passion of Our Lord and His most glorious Virgin Mother. Moreover, his work in defending the Christian faith and saving souls earned him universal admiration. His own writings provide a heaven-inspired exemplar and norm of the method of scholastic theology, which has been of immeasurable benefit to all theologians.

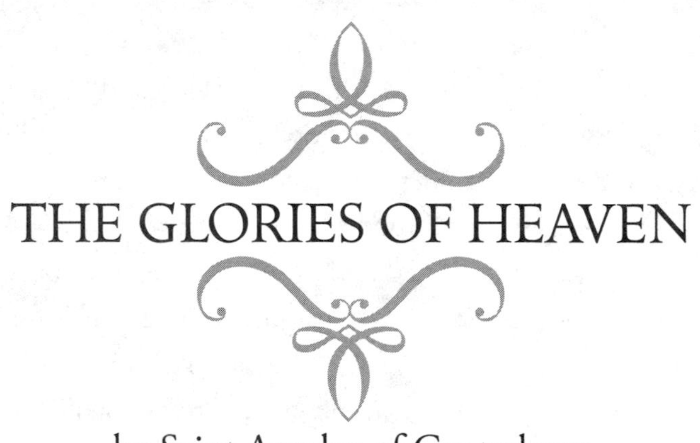

THE GLORIES OF HEAVEN

by Saint Anselm of Canterbury
and Eadmer of Canterbury

Eadmer's Introductory Letter to Brother William

To THE MOST reverend Sir, and my brother and friend of outstanding mercy, meekness, and honesty, William: I, Eadmer, the lowest and least of all the monks of the Church of Christ at Canterbury, wish you all the good things that God has promised to those who love Him.

You shall remember, I believe, that when our venerable father, Anselm, the archbishop of Canterbury, recently spent a few days at the monastery at Cluny,[1] he took the oppor-

[1] The abbey at Cluny, in east-central France, was a great monastic center at the time. It was especially known for the beauty of its liturgy

tunity to say a few words to the assembly of the brothers there. On that occasion, he said many wonderful things about the eternal happiness of the kingdom of heaven. And you, as you no doubt recall, requested that I should note down all that he said in the presence of the brothers at that time and give you a copy for your perusal and edification.

As you know, I am always eager to fulfill your wishes, and so I at once commenced this work. In the beginning, I had estimated it to be an easy and straightforward task, but it has proved, alas, to be rather more difficult than I expected! But my esteem and affection for you has compelled me to continue with the work I had begun, although, indeed, it may have been better had I not done so. For the material spoken by our father Anselm was beautiful and sublime, and yet I am an unskillful and inept scribe, and scarcely worthy or qualified to commit such things to writing.

It may therefore well be that my incompetence as a scribe will offend the reader more than the noble thoughts contained herein shall please them. What was wonderful and delightful to hear when spoken by Anselm may prove tedious and contemptible when written down by myself. But what I have committed to paper here has been done out of no other reason than sincere devotion and obedience, and motivated by the desire that the wonderful words which

---

and the cultivation of scholarship amongst its monks.

our venerable father, Anselm, spoke on that occasion may be faithfully recorded for yourself and for other readers.

Stay well, and please pray for me.

Eadmer

Anselm's Prologue

Many people, including quite a few of irreproachable morals and righteous deeds, who have cast off the vanities of this wicked world often ask: What is the reward which awaits us for living a good life? They may be answered appropriately with the words of Scripture, that their recompense shall be "what eye has not seen, nor ear heard, nor the mortal mind conceived—all that God has prepared for those who love him!"[2]

But for those who are unable to grasp the mysterious significance of this holy utterance, the same answer may be offered in different words: the reward due to those who serve God faithfully in this life is a future life, which lies beyond this world of time and space. This is an eternal life of everlasting joy and of endless bliss. It is a state in which all desires of the soul are fully satisfied and in which no longings go unfulfilled. This future eternal life will be one in which all possible good things shall be enjoyed in the highest degree of perfection.

---

[2] 1 Corinthians 2:9.

But such a description is not comprehensible or helpful to some. For they cannot imagine a state in which all the desires of the heart are perfectly satisfied, nor can they imagine the fulfillment of all the soul's desires, or the nature of the "highest possible good." For this reason, the description of the life of heaven which we have just offered may well seem to some to be unappealing and insipid.

What is to be said to such persons who find no delight in such a correct but philosophical description of the joys of paradise? In what way are they to be motivated towards good works?

It is my belief that they are to be handled in the same manner in which one feeds a young child. For if an enormous apple is given to such a child, they will be reluctant to eat it, as their small teeth and tender palate are not capable of handling such a fruit comfortably or with any pleasure. Rather, it is necessary to cut the apple up into small and digestible portions, and perhaps to soften it or sweeten it. Then they shall be able to consume the fruit easily and with true delight.

In the same way, we shall here endeavor to divide the mystery of the beatitude of eternal life into a series of smaller, comprehensible portions. If we consider each of the elements and qualities which the human mind naturally loves during this life, we are able to extrapolate and conjecture from these something of the nature of the future life. For in this future and unending life (which we shall attain if we hold fast to the commandments of God as we navigate our course through the perils of our earthly existence), all the good things which we currently desire or experience will be given to us in a much more excellent degree, in their very plentitude and perfection.

Such will be the approach we shall take as we embark upon our present discourse. Firstly, we shall consider those properties which pertain to the physical body, and which all human beings naturally desire and love. These include beauty, velocity, strength, freedom, well-being, pleasure, and longevity or immortality. Following this, we shall consider the good things which pertain to the life of the mind or the soul, and which, similarly, are naturally desired by all: wisdom, friendship, concord, power, honor, security, and joy. Finally, the pains and torments of the damned shall be briefly outlined and described.

Of course, there are those amongst the servants of God who, during this present life, deliberately deny themselves some of the good things enumerated above with the greatest conscientiousness. For example, those who are committed to a life of chastity seek neither physical beauty nor pleasure. But they do this not because they have no natural desire or love for such things. Rather, they prefer to renounce these particular good things in this passing world so that they may please God more, and thus attain them more fully in the life to come. Indeed, the good things of this present life—if one knows for certain that they do not offend God and do not impair one's love for that which is eternal—are always to be preferred to their contraries. This is obvious to our human nature itself.

Having offered these few prefatory remarks, let us now proceed to our consideration of the wonderful and marvelous happiness of the life of heaven, which—by the grace of God—we shall enjoy after the future resurrection of our bodies.

The Beauty of the Bodies of the Blessed

Beauty is a property which is naturally loved and desired by all. In the future life, the beauty of the resurrected bodies of the blessed shall be like the beauty of the sun, or rather shall be seven times more magnificent than that greatest of all celestial lights! For Scripture declares, "The just shall shine like the sun in the presence of God."[3]

The glorified body of the Lord Himself shall, of course, be infinitely more radiant than the sun, as no one could possibly doubt. Yet Saint Paul testifies that our own bodies will be like that of Christ when he writes, "He shall transform the body of our lowliness into the likeness of his own

[3] Matthew 13:43.

glorious body."[4] And Paul speaks with an authority that none would dare to question or contradict.

If there are any who are not satisfied with the evidence of Scripture but wish for a proof based on reason, I believe it may easily be shown that the bodies of the saints in heaven shall exceed the sun in beauty. For it is known that those who attain heaven become a temple and a throne of the Divinity and will be suffused with the glory of God and illuminated by His radiance. And yet the visible sun, as splendid as it is, is a mere created object, and it is therefore certainly less radiant than the divine splendor and less beautiful than the glory of the God Who fashioned it. It consequently follows that the bodies of the saints—suffused with this glory of God—will surpass the beauty and radiance of the sun itself.

The Velocity of the Glorified Bodies of the Saints in Heaven

VELOCITY IS A property which is loved and admired no less than beauty. When we arrive in our heavenly homeland, we shall possess a velocity and rapidity of motion which shall equal that of the angels, who move from heaven to earth and earth to heaven more quickly than one may say it.

[4] Philippian 3:32.

If anyone should consider it necessary to prove the rapidity and velocity of the angels, there is the well-known story of a certain human being [the prophet Habakkuk] who, when he was still weighed down by an earthly body, was carried by an angel from the land of Judea to the region of the Chaldeans. He carried with him food there [which he gave to Daniel in the lion's den] and was then transported back. And all of this took place instantaneously, as it were.[5]

In heaven, our own rapidity of movement will be fully comparable to that of the angels demonstrated in the above incident. For we are promised that in all respects we shall be made the equals of the angels of God. Indeed, the apostle Paul writes that even if our mortal bodies have been destroyed, dismembered, and dispersed in various locations throughout the earth, they shall, on the day of Final Judgment, be resurrected "in the twinkling of an eye."[6] In this expression, he provides eloquent testimony to the velocity with which our future incorruptible bodies shall be imbued. "That which is corruptible", he says, "shall put on incorruptibility; that which is mortal shall be clothed with immortality."[7]

We may perceive an example of such celestial velocity in the rays of the sun. Within a mere instant, these rays

[5] This incident is related in Daniel 14:33–39.
[6] 1 Corinthian 15:52.
[7] 1 Corinthians 15:53–54.

traverse the entire expanse of the firmament, from the most eastern point to the distant western horizon. From this plainly visible reality, it is easily inferred that the velocity which we have described is by no means impossible. Indeed, the rays of the sun are mere inanimate things, and yet they incontestably possess such marvelous speed. And animate things are, by their very nature, more rapid than inanimate things—so how much greater shall the velocity of the blessed be than that of the rays of the sun!

In fact, each of us already possesses something whose rapidity equals the rays of the sun, even within our earthly condition. For the rays of our eyes can reach the furthest corners of the distant skies and from thence return to themselves, all within the moment of time it takes to open and close our eyelids.[8] How much more must it be for the souls of the saints, who abide in the purest atmosphere of the heavens! And these souls, although already in paradise, do not yet enjoy the fullness of bliss, which shall happen only after the Final Judgment and the resurrection of the bodies of all the deceased.

When that happens, and the souls of the saints are reunited with their glorified, resurrected bodies, there shall be nothing more which they could possibly desire. Hence

---

[8] During the Middle Ages, it was believed that seeing occurred by means of the eyes sending forth rays, which went out, reflected off objects, and then returned to the eyes.

it follows that the soul which has been reunited with its resurrected body must possess mastery of the utmost velocity imaginable, equal to or surpassing that of the rays of the sun or of the eyes, or even of an incorporeal soul or angel.

The Immensity of the Strength of Those in Heaven

After beauty and velocity, we may consider strength as the next desirable quality, which shall be enjoyed in its perfection in heaven. It is obvious that all beings naturally prefer to be endowed with strength than to suffer from weakness and infirmity. For all those who attain the state of heaven and merit to be numbered amongst the citizens of the celestial Jerusalem, they shall possess such immense strength and power that nothing shall be able to prevent them from performing anything they wish. And there will be no force which is able to remove or overturn them from their state of eternal bliss in the love of God. And they will be able to employ the enormous strength which has been granted to them with no more effort than it currently takes us to blink our eyes!

Let no one be surprised or astonished by this. For in heaven, we shall be truly like the angels. Whatever the angels are able to do, we also shall be able to do. I firmly believe that there is no sane person who would believe that the holy angels do not possess the strength to do whatever they wish to do. Indeed, since the will of the holy angels and saints accords perfectly with the will of God in all matters, it follows that whatsoever they wish shall always be accomplished in accordance with the indisputable omnipotence of God.

But perhaps someone may object, saying that since in eternal life there is no change or alteration, there will be no action, and hence there will be no need or opportunity to exercise such strength. This is true. But we would offer a simple reply to such people. It is well known that in this mortal life a person may possess strength and abilities without ever actually bringing them into action, and a person may possess knowledge or skill without always making use of such knowledge or skill. In the same way, in heaven, we shall have at our disposal vast reserves of strength and power, even if there is no need to put them into action. For the very possession of the capacity will itself be pleasing and the source of exultation, even in the state of unchanging eternity.

This same observation applies with regard to the matter of velocity, previously discussed, and any other such qualities. If anyone objects that certain qualities (such as strength or velocity) have no possible applicability within the timeless and changeless realm of the celestial paradise, we respond that there is a joy and exultation simply in the possession of such qualities, which is not by any means dependent upon their active use.

The Unimpaired Freedom of the Saints in Heaven

Next, following the order we have proposed, we shall proceed to consider the perfect and unimpaired freedom enjoyed by the saints in heaven. Freedom is loved and esteemed no less by the celestial spirits and the souls of the blessed than it is valued and desired by we mortal human beings. Since we shall be endowed with the similitude of the angels when we are in heaven, we shall enjoy a liberty which is similar to theirs in every respect.

There is absolutely nothing which is able to constrain or restrict the holy angels. Rather, as has been noted, they are able to do all things in accordance with their will. This will, of course, is always in perfect harmony and agreement with the will of God Himself. So the unfettered liberty of the angels is a reflection of the perfect and transcendent liberty of God.

Similarly, in heaven, we shall encounter no obstacles or restrictions whatsoever. There shall be no enclosure which is able to detain us, nor any restraint which is able to obstruct us. In a similar way, the body of the Lord, after His resurrection, could not be held by the tomb. After His rising from the dead, He was able to pass through walls and closed doors with perfect freedom. And, as Saint Paul testifies, our own bodies shall be conformed to His. How great and utterly unfettered, then, shall be the liberty and freedom in which we shall rejoice within the celestial paradise!

The Perfect Well-Being of the Souls in Heaven

We may truly say that well-being is something which is loved and desired by all human beings. And concerning this condition of well-being, what may be said which is better or more true than that which the Psalmist declares that "the well-being[9] of the just comes from the Lord"?[10] And to those to whom the Lord gives this gift of well-being, what illness or infirmity could possibly prevail against them? Yet I do not see what I could offer as an adequate example or illustration of the well-being which we shall possess in heaven. For I perceive nothing like it in myself, nor in anybody else who dwells within this mortal flesh, which is comparable to the condition of perfect and unassailable well-being and health which we shall possess in the next world.

In this present time, we often believe that we are perfectly well when we do not consciously sense any particular pain. But we are deceiving ourselves in thinking this way. For often some part of our body may be injured or impaired, but we are not aware of this injury until something specifically aggravates or agitates it.

And for those who believe themselves to be completely well and in perfect health, how can we test whether this is

---

[9] The Latin word here, *salus*, is often translated as "salvation" or "help," but a more literal meaning is "health" or "well-being." Since this matches better with the sense of the text, "well-being" has been chosen here.

[10] Psalm 36:39.

really true? Take any apparently healthy and sound human body, whose possessor considers themselves to be in a condition of perfect well-being. Now, if you apply particular pressure to any part of that body or strike it with any degree of force, immediately the person will exclaim, "Stop that! You're hurting me." And did they not declare themselves to be in a state of perfect well-being just a moment before? But as soon as a little pressure is applied to them, they experience pain or annoyance. Do you believe that the state which they are in may be called well-being if it may so readily become suffering? I think not!

Thus, the present fragile condition which we describe as "health," yet which is still liable to pain, cannot be compared to the state of well-being which the Lord has promised us in the future. As Scripture declares, "God shall wash away every tear from their eyes, and there shall be no mourning or weeping, nor any pain, for the previous things have passed away."[11] And again, "They shall not hunger nor thirst anymore, nor shall the burning sun with its scorching heat fall upon them."[12] And, "God shall protect them with his right hand and shall defend them with his holy arm."[13]

What could possibly be able to harm those whom the right hand of God thus protects? I know that neither I

[11] Revelation 21:34.

[12] Isaiah 49:10. Revelation 7:16.

[13] Wisdom 5:2, 7.

myself nor anyone else in this mortal life has ever experienced firsthand the type of well-being which God shall give in heaven. This well-being will be completely unassailable and secure. If anyone were to ask me about a fever or any other kind of illness, I could easily offer an intelligent and informed answer, for I have either experienced such illnesses myself or have received information from other people who have experienced them. But as far as what I have never experienced myself, or never conversed with those who have experienced them—such as the perfect well-being of souls in heaven—I am unable to give an answer in the same way. Rather I find myself lacking both the knowledge and words to form any adequate description.

Nevertheless, I firmly and unhesitatingly believe that the well-being which we shall enjoy in the future world shall be, by its very nature, utterly unchangeable and inviolable. It shall surely saturate one's whole person with an ineffable sweetness, enchanting each one of the senses with unspeakable delight.

And anything which could cause the slightest trace of harm, impairment, or alteration to this state of perfect health will be far removed from it—and, indeed, absent altogether. For any such thing would be foreign to and incompatible with the immutability and eternity of the immortal God Who graciously bestows it. Although we cannot now fully imagine this condition of celestial well-being, its reality and attributes—comprising perfection, completeness, and changelessness—may be known with full confidence, since they are demonstrable by reason itself.

The Pleasures of Heaven

Following the order which we have set ourselves, we shall next discuss pleasure. We call "pleasure" all of those things which cause delight to the physical senses. And these are certainly loved and desired by all human beings. For each of the physical senses naturally strives after and yearns for those things which bring it delight or comfort. As examples of this, the sense of smell takes pleasure in sweet and rare fragrances, and the sense of taste enjoys experiencing fine flavors. Each of the other senses—sight, vision, and touch—is similarly attracted to those things which correspond to its capacities and propensities and cause it delight. The attractions to those things which delight the senses are what constitute the natural appetites of the human being.

Yet such delights will not *always* bring delight, and such pleasures will not *forever* bring pleasure. For after a certain period, even those who love them most will encounter a feeling of satiety, and then boredom or revulsion. For, by their very nature, their capacity to satisfy is transitory, and they appeal to the merely animal part of our nature. Yet those pleasures which the just shall enjoy to the full in the world to come will be everlasting. They shall appeal not to the lower physical senses only but also to the higher mental and spiritual faculties. Since they are so different from our present pleasures, I cannot see how anyone can learn what the delights of heaven will really be like. For nothing that we experience here on earth could ever suffice to give us an example of their nature.

The pleasures we will possess in heaven are of such a kind that the more they are experienced, the more fervently shall one desire them. For, since they are perfect in nature, they shall bring satisfaction and yet never give rise to any boredom or tedium. I believe that there is no one living, or no one who has ever lived, who would not prefer the taste and experience of these perfect heavenly delights than any earthly pleasure whatsoever!

There are two forms of beatitude, and similarly two forms of misery. One of these forms of beatitude is greater and one is lesser. Similarly, one of the forms of misery is greater and the other is lesser. The greater beatitude is that which is enjoyed by the angels and souls of the blessed in the kingdom of God. The lesser beatitude was the happiness which was experienced in the garden of Eden, the earthly paradise in which Adam was first located.

The greater of the miseries is that of the eternal fires of hell. The lesser of the miseries consists in the sufferings and tribulations which we incessantly undergo in this passing mortal life.

None of us have ever experienced either the greater or the lesser form of beatitude since we have never dwelt either in the kingdom of heaven nor in the garden of Eden. But if we *had* experienced the lesser beatitude—that is the earthly paradise—perhaps through this we would be able to imagine the pleasures of the greater beatitude of heaven. All of us have experienced the lesser from of misery—that is, the sufferings of this earthly exile—into which we were all born and have been raised and now dwell. And, on the basis of these present miseries, we can fairly easily imagine the greater miseries of hell, and can easily speak of them and explicate them whenever we wish.

It is to be noted, though, that the pleasure of heaven of which we now speak is merely one portion of the greater beatitude of the kingdom of God. I do not see how I can try to explain this except perhaps through a similitude based on the opposite phenomenon—that is, pain. Imagine in your mind a human being, and then imagine that burning, red-hot irons are applied to the pupils of his eyes and to his other members. Think of the great pain he will experience—how agony shall suffuse his whole body so that neither the marrow of his bones nor his intestines nor any part of him shall be free from the most extreme discomfort. How could we describe the condition of such a person? He is thoroughly tormented; he will be completely filled with agony and utterly overcome with anguish.

In a similar, but opposite, way, in the future life of heaven, ineffable pleasure shall completely inebriate and saturate those who are saved. An unimaginable outflowing of delight shall fill them and all their senses with the most indescribable sweetness. The eyes, the ears, the nostrils, the mouth, the hands, the feet, the throat, the heart, the loins, the lungs, the bones, and even the very marrow of the bones shall all experience the plentitude of ecstasy. Each of the senses and parts of the body shall enjoy this plenitude individually, and also all of the senses and the whole body will enjoy it in its supreme totality. This delight of the senses shall be of a miraculous sweetness and marvelous delight, such that the entire human being will drink deeply from the crystalline stream of celestial pleasure and be utterly and gloriously inebriated by its all-surpassing fullness![14]

The Immortality of the Life of Heaven

For those who have attained all the good things described up to this point in our discourse, I cannot imagine what more they could possibly desire, as far as comfort, power, well-being, and pleasure of the body are concerned. Yet there still remains one more thing to which human beings

[14] Cf. Psalm 35:9.

naturally aspire, and that is length of life. Even during our difficult earthly existence, human beings desire longevity and to reach the fullness of years.

For the blessed souls in heaven, such longevity will be given in its most complete and perfect form—which is to say, extending to a life without end or close. For Scripture declares quite clearly that "the just shall live forever."[15]

***

Apart from all the things which we have enumerated so far, there are still other benefits and boons which are naturally loved and desired by human beings. Those things which we have discussed already—beauty, velocity, strength, freedom, well-being, pleasure, and longevity or immortality—pertain primarily to the physical body. But the other things which are loved and desired by human beings relate to the soul. These are likewise seven in number, and they bring delight to the mind and heart no less than those good things we have already described delight and satisfy the body. These desirable properties and conditions which pertain to the soul are: wisdom, friendship, concord, power, honor, safety, and joy. Each of these shall be considered in the next section of our treatise.

---

[15] Wisdom 5:16.

Wisdom

Wisdom is something which we all naturally value, desire, and seek in this present life. Yet our wisdom in this present life, even for the most learned and astute of people, is always partial, fragmentary, and uncertain. But in the next life, the blessed souls in heaven shall possess wisdom which is of such a wonderful extent that there shall be absolutely nothing which they do not know or understand. For God shall permit and cause them to know everything which can be known, including all things past, present, and future.

In the kingdom of heaven, each shall know everything, and everyone and everything shall be perfectly known. There will be nothing which remains concealed, neither what homeland nor what people nor what family anyone has originated from nor what deeds anyone has done during the course of their earthly life.

But perhaps someone will be concerned when they hear this. "What?!" they may object, "Will all the sins I have committed while I was alive be known to all? Surely, if I have confessed them to a priest, they are entirely deleted and shall be completely forgotten in heaven!" Here, you speak well. But when you have entered the glory of heaven you shall be purged of all the culpability, shame, and guilt for your sins. And, as you stand before the face of God, it would surely be a mark of ingratitude for you not to have in your mind just how much mercy God has shown you and how many sins He has forgiven you? And how could you possibly give thanks to God for forgiving your sins unless some memory of them remains with you? Therefore, so that you may eternally thank God for His mercy to you, I believe that you will need to recall how great this mercy has actually been. And so the memory of sins, and their forgiveness, will necessarily remain.

Thus everything that is in the conscience of each blessed soul—including the sins which have been committed and forgiven—shall be known and clearly revealed to every other blessed soul. But this shall not be the source of any shame or confusion. On the contrary, it will then be the cause both of giving glory and thanks to God and a source of true joy and delight to the soul which has received the mercy of God.

Certainly, once you have attained the glory of heaven, any sins you had committed during your earthly life will no longer be a source of anxiety to your conscience, nor shall they oppress your heart with any sense of guilt or shame. The situation will be similar to that of a person who has once suffered wounds, which are later perfectly healed. The former wounds no longer cause that person any discomfort, though the visible scars may remain. Or it may perhaps be compared to the condition of a person who has reached venerable and respectable old age; such a person will normally not feel the slightest shame about the foibles and misdeeds they may have committed while they were still in their infancy or youth.

Once you have attained the kingdom of heaven, the perfect well-being, stainless purity, complete remission, and unassailable impunity which you have secured will fill you with perfect joy. Thoughts of the sins you committed during your earthly life, once they have been forgiven, shall not cause you any more fear or anxiety than Saint Peter now suffers from the fact that he once denied Christ, or that Saint Paul now suffers because he once persecuted the Church, or which Saint Mary Magdalene now suffers for her former sins. For each of these saints knows with perfect certainty that their sins, though perhaps many and serious, are now entirely forgiven.

Indeed, through former sins which have been forgiven—just like an illness which has been successfully cured—the mercy, power, and wisdom of the divine Physician is revealed. And by this means, the virtues of the Physician Who healed the afflictions and illness become all the more exuberantly admired, praised, and glorified. If you consider the matter rightly, the praise and honor given to the Physician—Who, in this case, is God Himself—shall also be your own glory.

But you might say, "Certainly, I agree that the praise of God will be my glory! But there will be so many there who, in comparison to me, will be almost completely innocent. These, if they had knowledge of all my former sins and all my shameful acts, will be filled with shock and horror. They shall not be able to refrain from judging me! For there is a reward which befits the righteous and a retribution which is due to the guilty—such as myself."

My anxious brother or sister, in this matter you need have no fear! For things will be completely different to how you are now imagining them. For most of those whom you now believe to be so innocent and so free from sins in their earthly life, you will then find that, just like you, they have committed their own particular sins and have struggled with their own weaknesses and temptations. And they shall realize that by sinning, you have offended God alone. And when they see that God Himself has completely forgiven your offences and entirely cancelled your debts, there shall be no reason why they should presume to judge or condemn you. Indeed, they shall realize that for themselves to judge you when God has forgiven you would be to offend and contradict God. Rather, they shall more deeply marvel at the ineffable and infinite mercy of God—not only exhibited towards you, but also to themselves. This wondrous mercy was shown through you since God so graciously rescued you from the pit of iniquity into which you had slipped. But—if they have been lesser sinners during their earthly life—they will also appreciate that it is only by the same mercy of God that they themselves did not fall into similar depths of sin. They will praise and glorify the Lord, that it was His fortitude and aid which permitted you to escape safely from the whirlpool of wickedness in which you had found yourself. And they shall realize that it was divine Grace alone which prevented them from tumbling into this same whirlpool from which, perhaps, they (unlike you) would not have escaped.

In heaven, you will see no shame whatsoever attached to the revelation of your former sins. Rather, the fact that they have been forgiven will be the source of endless praise and gratitude. The angels themselves shall welcome you into their company. And if anyone should presume to judge you as being unworthy of this on the basis of your past actions, you shall have a sure and just means of defending yourself against such persons. "And what is that?" you may ask. Listen carefully, and I shall tell you.

Imagine for yourself a certain one of the angels who stands before you and says, "You, O offspring of Adam, are made of dust and ashes, and you were, by your very nature, destined to return to the same dust. And yet you rebelled against the God Who created you. Acting against His precepts, you threw yourself into the filth of sin, while swollen up with pride and impurity. And now you seek to be similar to us holy angels, who never once deviated from the will of God!"

To this you may respond, "If, as you say, I am fashioned from dust and ash, it is hardly surprising that I have, in the past, slipped into the dirt of sin. Yet once I came to know the mercy of Christ, I tried always to spurn those things which I knew displeased Him. And I earnestly endeavored to do those things which accorded with His will. For this reason, I underwent many tribulations and deprivations—including hunger, thirst, vigils, penances, humiliations, and innumerable other trials. I endured all this for the honor of Christ, and I came to consider all earthly things as nothing. Through each of the hardships and austerities I accepted and sustained, I sought nothing but to be reconciled with God!

"But, you angels, what have *you* ever endured? For you have always been in a state of glory and innocence, and you have always known the bliss of the presence of the Lord. The right hand of God has constantly kept you safe from all the attacks and temptations of sin so that no stain of guilt has ever once polluted you. And the fact that you have never been attacked by temptation nor ever fallen is due purely to the grace of God."

Now, the response we have proposed above is well suited for those who have committed grave sins in their life and then repented—that is to say, for those who have "entered the kingdom of heaven by violence,"[16] so to speak. But for

[16] Matthew 11:12.

those who entered the kingdom in another way, the following answer will serve them well: "Truly, it is Christ Himself who has paid the price of human sin. For our sake, He deigned to become human, to suffer, and to die. He poured out His most precious blood in order to render us worthy consorts of the kingdom of heaven! And is not His divine blood capable of easily achieving this thing? Is it not so powerful as to be able even to make us wretched and sinful mortals into perfect beings and to bring about our salvation?"

How will the angels in heaven reply to this? Surely, since they are essentially good and therefore wish always to acquiesce to truth and reason, they shall declare that the outpouring of Christ's blood indeed *does* suffice to render sinful human beings perfect. Thus they will acknowledge you as their rightful companion and peer. And if even the holy angels do this, how much more shall all other human beings also do so, including those whom you consider to have been more innocent than yourself? They will all joyously accept you and honor you on account of the sublime truth of your salvation through God's mercy.

The wisdom which we shall possess in heaven is of the nature we have described. Consider, you who hear me, how wonderful it shall be! By it, you will know all things about all others, just as all others shall know all things about you. [And this knowledge and insight shall serve to glorify the

Lord and to reveal the depths of His mercy and power all the more magnificently!][17]

The Wonderful Friendship amongst the Souls in Heaven

Does it not follow from the wisdom described in the previous chapter [whereby all will know and understand each other perfectly], that a certain marvelous and all-encompassing friendship shall prevail amongst the souls in heaven? By means of this unitive and unanimous friendship, each will embrace the other with sincere fervor of love.

For I cannot see how it should be otherwise, since all are members of the very same body of Christ. And Christ, Who Himself is our peace,[18] shall be the one head of all. In the same way that no members of a body, even the lesser ones, are not truly loved by the body itself and all the other members which comprise it, even so will all the souls in the kingdom of heaven be united in affection and perfect solidarity.

You will love all your heavenly companions just as they will all love you. Consider how much love and friendship

---

[17] This final paragraph, and the latter portion of the previous one, includes several apparent textual errors and corruptions. The translation offered here restores what seems to be the intended sense.

[18] Cf. Ephesians 2:14.

you shall thus enjoy in the shared possession of that glorious kingdom of eternal joy and peace!

Nevertheless, let us pass from the friendship which will exist among the souls of the blessed and contemplate now another good thing which shall come to you in that future life in heaven. For there will be One Who loves you more than you love yourself, and more than all the other blessed beings combined could possibly love you. And you also shall love this One—Who is God Himself—more than you love all others and more than you love yourself. And that divine love will be of a sweetness that exceeds all description and a delight which transcends all comprehension!

Concord

It is known that even among people who sincerely love each other, disagreements and differences are apt to spring up from time to time. One person sees things in one way, while another views them in another. One desires what another flees from, and *vice versa.* For this reason, it is pertinent to add to our enumeration of the good things of heaven the fact that as well as universal love and friendship, there will also be universal concord or agreement. For without this concord, there would be a certain impairment of, or blemish upon, the perfect goodness and peace which shall there prevail.

There will indeed be such concord and unanimity there that you shall never sense anyone who differs in the least from what you will yourself. We shall all truly be one Body, one Church, and one Spouse of Christ. There will be no more discord than there is between the different members of the same body. Just as you will observe in the motion of your eyes, whenever you turn one eye to look in a particular direction the other eye automatically turns its gaze in the same direction, so shall the will of all those in heaven be united in the same intention, without any discrepancy whatsoever.

But perhaps you may ask, "What shall be this will and intention which all have in common?" It shall be the will of God itself. For your own will shall be in precise accordance with God's will, and of all other blessed souls who are similarly united to God. Is it possible for the head to desire one thing while the other members of the body desire something different? [Certainly not!]

But here, perhaps someone may secretly complain in their heart, saying, "If God and all the assembly of the blessed shall desire exactly the same things which I desire, then they shall also desire an increase in my status and glory! For I myself should hardly be able to prevent myself from desiring that. Indeed, I should aspire to be amongst the very greatest in heaven!"

To this I respond that if anyone there desired to be equal to Saint Peter himself in glory, he should be! He should be equal *in glory*, I say, but he would not be identical to Peter *in person.* For if he wished to be identical to Saint Peter *in person*, that would mean that he would then no longer desire to be himself—or, in other words, he should desire not to exist. But this is, by its very nature, impossible for the souls of the blessed.

Furthermore, it is also impossible for one of the souls in heaven to seek to be equal to Saint Peter in glory unless he is equal in merit. For there will be a beautiful harmony which prevails within the celestial body of Christ, which is made up of the souls in heaven. And no member of this body shall desire to compromise or disturb this harmony. For in a human body, the foot does not aspire to attain the position of the hand, nor does the hand desire to perform the function of a foot. Neither does the mouth or nose seek to be where the eyes are; nor do the eyes wish to leave their sockets and take up the position of the mouth or the nose. And if they *were* transferred, it would be a grievous affliction for them! In the same way, there is a wonderful and glorious disposition of all things in the blessed city of God so that each member loves most his own allotted position within it and never desires to exchange it for another's rank or status.

"Why is this?" you may ask. The answer is that it is because to each and every soul, its own happiness and blessedness will be perfectly sufficient. For if any soul desired to attain a place within the body of Christ which was different or greater than what it actually possessed, that would necessarily mean that it felt that something was absent from it, and that it was not yet perfectly happy, but still experienced the sorrow of some unfulfilled desire. But in the wonderful kingdom of heaven, all sorrow, all unfulfilled desire, shall be completely absent! Therefore, each soul shall be perfectly content and perfectly fulfilled, and unanimous and undisturbed concord will prevail forever over all.

Power

FOR ALL SOULS who have attained entrance into the kingdom of heaven, their will shall always be in perfect accord with the will of God Himself. They shall want everything that God wants and not wish for anything which God does not want. Now, if your own will is identical to the will of God, it necessarily follows that there can be nothing which you desire which you are not able to attain. In this regard, you shall share in the omnipotence of God, since whatever He wills (which will be exactly the same as what you will) is done; thus you shall be, effectively, omnipotent yourself!

Honor

Since such immense power will be yours when you have entered the kingdom of heaven, commensurate honor shall also certainly not be lacking.

Let us consider for a brief moment what *honor* exactly is. Imagine a certain poor and wretched beggar, from whom all solace is absent, and who is afflicted with hideous ulcers and other foul wounds and infirmities. This poor beggar does not even possess a cloak to shield himself from the bitter cold of winter. Now imagine that a most powerful and magnificent king is passing by and happens to see this poor wretch lying in the dirt by the wayside. And the king feels pity and compassion for the poor man and commands that his wounds be treated and healed and that the beggar should be clothed in fine garments from his own stores. Moreover, the king determines and declares that he shall adopt the wretched beggar as his very own son, and he commands that henceforth all the subjects of his kingdom are to regard him as such. He orders that none are to oppose, disparage, or belittle his newly adopted son (despite the fact that he was formerly a beggar), and he even makes him heir of his entire kingdom, bestowing upon him an exalted title of royal dignity.

Would you not say that this man, who was once a wretched beggar but has been adopted and elevated by so great a king, has been magnificently honored? But this is certainly just what God, the King of the universe, has done for you! For we fallen human beings are born in the corruption of the flesh, and our lot is filled with many miseries. And, in the midst of our sorrows and suffering, we are bereft of all consolation and subject to all the turmoil and weakness of fleshly passions. And, although we are covered with the wounds of misery and the ulcers of sin, God Himself comes to our assistance, motivated by His mercy alone. He will cure us of our afflictions and—in the fullness of time—adorn us with the blessings of perfect righteousness and incorruptibility. He will adopt us as His sons and daughters through grace, and make us sharers in, and heirs to, the untold splendors of His glorious kingdom. He will establish us as peers and co-heirs with His only-begotten Son, and shall place all created things under our dominion.

And God will even command that we be called gods. For He has declared in the Sacred Scriptures, "You are gods, and all children of the Most High!"[19] It is God Himself Who will raise you to divinity. And if God makes you divine, you shall be divine indeed![20]

But perhaps some will object to this, saying, "That is all able to be applied to the great apostles and to the martyrs and other great and holy souls. But to me—I wish! Perhaps

[19] Psalm 81:6; John 10:34.
[20] Cf. John 8:36.

I shall manage to be counted as the least in the kingdom of heaven, but I could never possibly attain to the divine honor which you have described."

Listen and understand how this attaining to a divine state shall work, which God expresses in the words, "You are gods, and all children of the Most High."[21] So that the significance of these words may be better illustrated, consider, as an example, the nature of fire and the nature of things which are set alight by that fire. The fire is able to set alight other objects and to convey to them its fiery nature without suffering any diminishment of itself thereby. In the same way, the divine nature of God shall be shared with those souls who participate in the beatitude of heaven as if by inflaming them with the fire of God's own divinity.

The fire itself is one, and in its nature it is hot. If you place into this fire a piece of wood, a piece of lead, and a piece of iron together, see what shall happen! The wood shall be transformed into coals, and the lead shall very soon melt. These substances absorb the fire, and their nature becomes fiery. In the glowing coals, the radiant brightness of the fire is to be perceived, and in the molten lead, the intense heat of the flames is fully present. As for the iron, it does not change its form like the other substances, but nevertheless still absorbs into itself the heat of the fire—becoming hotter than either the burning coals from the wood or the

---

[21] Psalm 81:6; John 10:34.

molten lead. Each of the substances—the wood, the lead, and the iron—remains itself, yet becomes a participant in the nature of the fire and may be said to become a part of the fire.

Thus shall it be amongst the souls of the blessed in the heavenly realms. Some will be closer to the ineffable majesty of God, and it is of these that it may most pertinently be said, "You are gods."[22] But even those who occupy the lower ranks of the celestial court and are further removed from the throne of the Deity shall also participate in the divine nature according to their capacity and properties. They also may be referred to as "gods" since they will be participants in the nature of the one divinity.

Once you have obtained the blessing of such an exalted honor, I do not see how you could possibly wish for anything more. When you enjoy the magnificent glory which we have here described, shall this not be enough for you? "Certainly!" you will say.

Now, my friend, if you were granted all these stupendous and wonderful things which we have described for one day, would it make you happy? "Without doubt," you will reply. If you were to be given them to enjoy for a month, or for a year, would you then rejoice? I dare to say that if you were given them for such a time, your joy would be without measure.

---

[22] Psalm 81:6.

But you will have these things not for one day only, nor for a month, nor for a year, but for all eternity! You will possess them forever, for ages unending, and there will be no possible thing you could desire or imagine or wish for which will not be yours!

Absolute Security

If you were somehow able to be made completely secure with regards to all you now possess and enjoy in this earthly life—so that there was no way you could possibly lose them or be deprived of them—you would certainly feel great relief and exultation. But if this security pertained not merely to the limited and imperfect things of this earthly existence but also to the wonderful and perfect things of the eternal life of heaven so that you were sure of possessing and enjoying them forever with no possible danger of ever losing them, how greatly should you then rejoice?

I believe that the thought of such unassailable security must bring to you an immense jubilation of heart, knowing that you are to possess such unimaginably good things forever and ever. Indeed, how eagerly you should aspire to such a glorious state!

How could you possibly lose the good things of heaven once you have attained them? Either you would have to renounce them voluntarily, or God would have to take them away from you, or another being who was stronger than God would have to deprive you of them, contrary to the will of both God and yourself. But certainly you yourself would never wish to renounce the enjoyment of the perfect goodness and joy of heaven [since it is in the nature of every being to desire its own happiness]. Nor should God, Who had bestowed such blessings in His generous and merciful goodness, ever wish to deprive you of them, [for to do thus would be contrary to His own nature and will]. Nor is there any being who is stronger than God Who could possibly deprive you of the goodness of Heaven, contrary to the will of both God and yourself. You will therefore be perfectly and absolutely secure in your happiness and will have no need whatsoever to fear the incursion of any foe, adversity, or misfortune which could deprive you of anything which you possess or enjoy.

How great will your joy then be! For you will possess and enjoy with absolute and everlasting security all the things we have described thus far—the very perfection of beauty, velocity, pleasure, endless longevity, strength, freedom, health and well-being, wisdom, friendship, concord, power, honor, and security! Rather, you will enjoy forever a bliss and glory which is utterly beyond all human imagination and which exceeds anything that can be put into writing or into speech. This shall be the very consummation of all possible joys!

Indeed, I myself find that words fails me at this point in trying to describe the inestimable bliss of those who shall enjoy for endless ages this blessed happiness and happy blessedness. When you arrive in the kingdom of heaven, the splendid realm of inapproachable light, you shall enjoy all these things in perfection, and there shall be absolutely nothing in which you shall not rejoice!

Perfect Joy

If there is anyone whom you love just as much as you love yourself, you will rejoice in the happiness of that person just as much as you will rejoice in your own. So, if there was such a person who possessed blessings and joys which were equal to your own, would not your own happiness be thereby doubled? Would it not be the case that if there were two, or even more, whom you loved just as much as yourself, your own happiness would increase when you perceived that their own joys equaled yours?

If you recall what we have written about the universal and perfect friendship which shall redound in the kingdom of heaven, you will realize that you shall love all the other souls of the blessed as much as yourself, and they will likewise love you with an equal love. And there shall be there a thousand times a thousand souls who enjoy the perfection of happiness, or rather a thousand times a hundred thousand, or rather a number which is utterly incomprehensible and uncountable! And, [applying the principle we have just described], each one shall have their own joys multiplied in perceiving the joys of all the others.

This supreme joy, therefore, will be both inside and outside, joy above and joy below, joy surrounding the soul in every direction and in every aspect! And this, as we have said at the beginning of our discourse, is "what God has prepared for those who love him."[23] This is what, in my judgment, can be described—insofar as it is possible to be described—as eternal beatitude, eternal happiness, the perfect fullness of all possible comforts and delights, in which nothing at all shall be lacking. This is what all the friends of God will possess in the unending life to come! Nevertheless, we do not claim to have fully or adequately described it. For it is, to be sure, infinitely more than all we have managed to convey in our humble and simple words.

The Misery of Those Who Will Be Condemned

While the just shall enjoy such a supreme and overflowing abundance of happiness in the life to come, it remains to say that the unjust, on the contrary, shall be miserable with unimaginable sorrow. We have described the life of the blessed (insofar as we are able) as being, through the

[23] 1 Corinthians 2:9.

gift of God, suffused with miraculous beauty, limitless velocity, invincible strength, unfettered liberty, perfect health and well-being, as well as the highest degree of pleasure. And those who attain to this wonderful life shall rejoice in unimaginable and unending jubilation.

But, on the contrary, those who are deprived of this blessed state and condemned to eternal damnation shall experience an unimaginable foulness, sluggishness, weakness, stupor, and abject servitude. Unceasing languor and pain shall leave then mourning and wailing for all eternity. And the limitless duration of life, which the blessed shall receive with the greatest love on account of the felicity which they enjoy, shall be endured with the greatest odium by the damned on account of the untold miseries with which they are tormented.

As for wisdom, as has been noted, this shall be a source of profound joy and honor in the minds of all the souls in heaven. But for the wicked, whatever knowledge they possess shall become a source of regret or confusion. As has been noted, there shall be a chaste and unwavering friendship which unites all those who have attained to the kingdom of God so that they are united in perfect peace and the most harmonious concord. But if there is any unity or fellowship amongst the damned, it shall only be through the fact that they share in torments and are fellow sufferers. However much more such persons may feel affection towards each other, so much more shall their pains be increased, as they witness those to whom they feel sympathy also suffering. But, on the contrary, there will be no genuine love or harmony amongst such unfortunate and condemned beings at all. For they shall be in continual discord and conflict with all creatures, and all creatures shall likewise be in conflict with them.

And—in contrast to the plenitude of power which will be enjoyed by all those in heaven—those who find themselves in the realms of eternal suffering shall find themselves utterly without power. They will be continually frustrated in all their efforts, endeavors, desires, and wishes. For they shall be able to do or possess nothing which they desire, but, on the contrary, whatever they do *not* want shall befall them. And instead of the immense honor which the saints shall possess, the souls of those condemned shall be afflicted with unrelieved shame and disgrace.

And shall there be any end to their state of woe, you ask? Alas, no! Just as those in heaven will feel their happiness augmented by the knowledge that they are absolutely sure that it shall last forever, so those who have made themselves enemies of God will despair when they realize that their torments shall never reach an end. Instead of the timeless and ineffable joy which the just shall receive in heaven, those who have—through their wicked works and lack of repentance—made themselves the companions of demons shall inherit unimaginable sorrows without end or relief.

Having considered all of these things, it is very easy to see how useful and profitable it is for a person to spend their earthly lives in the eager performance of works of justice and righteousness and the cultivation of good morals. Conversely, it is plain how dangerous and foolish a thing it is to neglect good deeds during this life and to become enmeshed in vice and iniquity. For one is a path to unlimited and everlasting joy, whereas the other leads to unspeakable miseries which go on forever and ever!

We may consider the matter more broadly—that is, how useful and profitable it is for a person to live a righteous life and to cultivate a good character, and thus to win final admittance into the kingdom of heaven. For it is useful not only to the person concerned (insofar as it leads to their tranquility in the present life and their eternal happiness in the next), but it is pleasing also to God Himself, and to the holy angels. Indeed, the cultivation of personal virtue and goodness is useful, profitable, and pleasing also to our fellow human beings and to all of creation!

Firstly, it is pleasing to God. Of course, the actions of any created being cannot affect God's own perfect beatitude in the slightest, or be "useful" to Him in any way. For God is entirely self-sufficient. But rather, our good works help to build up the "City of God," which is constructed by the actions of all people who do what is right. This City of God comes into being through humans beings living in accordance with divine laws, and both glorifies God and promotes our own happiness and peace.

How human righteousness is pleasing to the holy angels can be understood by considering the rejoicing felt by a community of good people when one of their number who was missing is returned to them. In a similar way, when a good soul is admitted to the company of the angels in the celestial homeland, great joy abounds amongst them all. For the arrival of this priceless, immortal soul has helped to complete their destined number and to bring closer to perfection the glorious communion of the blessed in God's eternal court.

We have stated also that the goodness and virtue of any individual is useful and pleasing to all other good human beings and, indeed, to creation itself. For each good person is inflamed by an ardent desire for the eternal joys of heaven and must rejoice when they see the perfection of God's kingdom approaching more quickly. So in witnessing the good and virtuous actions of others and realizing that these other good people are similarly hastening towards the same heavenly homeland, they must experience genuine joy and satisfaction. And all of creation naturally strives for the perfection of the City of God, which is the final consummation of its own ultimate purpose. Creation itself therefore rejoices to see the soul of any good person make its way towards heaven, and finally to enter it. This entrance into heaven (following the death of a good person) is not experienced as a loss by the created world but rather is another step towards its own ultimate perfection, and hence the source of a profound joy.

How great a thing is this virtue and goodness which leads a soul to the eternal happiness of heaven! For each individual instance is an indispensable part of the pre-destined reparation of the entire cosmos and a precious component of the ultimate consummation of the celestial kingdom, the glorious bringing to perfection of God's universal plan. And truly, this divine plan will not be perfected until each and every individual soul who is destined to be saved shall have attained to eternal bliss and have entered into the number of the elect. The perfection and consummation of this ultimate good is necessarily delayed in this realm of time and space until the very last of the whole multitude of the elect will have reached heaven.

Thus God Himself, the holy angels, all blessed souls, and all of creation rejoice whenever a person advances towards heaven and eventually attains it. They desire this with a single, unanimous will, and all the denizens of heaven welcome each new fellow citizen and co-heir of their celestial kingdom with heartfelt and boundless exultation. For each new arrival contributes to the perfection of the City of God, and the eternally predestined number of the host of the blessed, comprising both the holy angels and the souls of the saints.

If such is the glory and joy which emerges from the salvation of any individual soul, we may gain an insight into what the situation will be for those who find themselves cut off from the kingdom of heaven by considering diametrically opposite conditions. Such people will be deprived of being part of this wonderful consummation of the City of God. They shall be definitely excluded from the number of the elect and from the exultant host of the saints and the angels. Now, each human being was created by God for the very purpose of enjoying this blessedness. Thus those who find themselves excluded for it shall realize that they have ignored the destiny which imbued ultimate meaning to their existence and have not become what they were created to be.

Any person will be naturally grieved and saddened when they lose something or someone whom they value. In an analogous way, God Himself shall grieve and be saddened by the loss of any human being whom He has created in His own glorious image. [In a manner of speaking,] God will mourn when He sees their soul being seized away from Him by the cunning and malignity of the wicked devil to undergo eternal torments and shame.[24] For this reason, a soul that is condemned to everlasting punishment is said to

[24] This image of God being grieved or saddened should be understood as a metaphoric and anthropomorphic manner of speaking since it clearly does not pertain to God's nature in an absolute sense, which is necessarily eternally and infinitely blessed and impassible.

be a "lost soul," for it has been lost to God, for whose kingdom and glory it was created. Instead of achieving its noble destiny, it will have been cast into the perpetual darkness and confusion of the devil and all his wretched companions.

Consider how truly wonderful is the beatitude of the eternal life which God offers to us! And as much as this eternal life is glorious, so much, on the contrary, will be the wretchedness and misery of unending death and torment which is the alternative. In order that we may flee with all urgency from the latter and seek with eager longing to acquire the former, it is useful to elaborate further on both—namely, on how the interminable pains of hell shall excruciate the wicked and how the unceasing happiness of heaven shall delight the good.

May those who are good preserve in their righteousness so that they may eventually come to enjoy the reward due to them! But may those who are wicked cease to be what they are so that, by ceasing to be wicked, they may escape from the torments which await them. Truly, goodness is like a radiant light and a clear brightness which illumines the path of those who aspire to it and those who adhere to it. By means of this light of goodness, they may walk with assurance and safety along the perilous and winding paths of this mortal life and, all the while, be fully cognizant of the blessings of the eternal life towards which they are journeying. Yet wickedness is, by its very nature, a profound darkness and a dense and shadowy gloom. Thus the one who follows the path of wickedness walks like one who is blinded or like a person staggering under the influence of drunkenness. Such a person does not perceive the terrible destination towards which they are steadily heading but rather stumbles into the pit of perdition wholly unaware and taken by surprise.

But perhaps there are sinners who are ashamed of their own wickedness and dread the end to which it must lead them and genuinely desire to turn from their former ways and to become good. The first thing that is necessary for such a sinner to do to avert disaster is to recognize their own sinfulness. To do this is to realize that they are enwrapped in darkness, insofar as their own judgment permits them. But—alas!—there are a great many who are so deeply shrouded in the darkness of sin that they are entirely unable to perceive this very darkness which surrounds and envelops them. Tragically, such people are typically entirely unable to comprehend fully the wretchedness of the bitter plight in which they languish.

On the Necessity of Self-Knowledge, Confession, and Humility[25]

The very first act of goodness for any person is, therefore, the humble willingness to recognize the state of his own

[25] This chapter division and heading is not in the original but has been added by the translator.

soul and the quality of his own life. The more deeply and honestly a person knows himself, the closer he is to the divine light of truth. If a person recognizes himself to be a sinner and wishes to become good, it behooves him first of all to mourn what he currently is. Otherwise, such a person is not speaking truly and sincerely in saying that he wishes to become good.

To the knowledge and honest recognition of one's own sinfulness, it is then necessary to add the sorrow of compunction and genuine repentance. Hence it is very wisely written in Sacred Scripture that, "The one who adds to knowledge, adds also to sorrow."[26] But this sorrow is not in itself sufficient, but requires appropriate medicine for its reparation and healing. It is therefore essential to reveal the sorrow and pain of the awareness of one's sin to a minister of the Church, who has the skill, expertise, and sacramental grace to cure the wound.

Indeed, horrid viruses and foul germs breed within all wounds which are concealed, and which become putrid and infected. Such a festering wound cannot be healed until it is opened up and exposed so that the filth and fetor which lies within it can be drained from it. That is how it is also with the wounds of sin when they are concealed and covered up. Until they are exposed to the light through honest confession, they cannot be healed. For the wound

[26] Ecclesiastes 1:18.

must be opened and cleaned, and its lethal foulness must be washed away. Only then can the healing medicine of penitence exercise its proper effect.

A person should not be afraid of the possibility of human tongues saying ill things about them. Nor should they be cowardly in accepting the medicine of penance, which alone can heal them. For if they are ashamed and embarrassed because a few mortal beings may know their sins and gossip about them, how shall they possibly withstand having all their evil deeds and thoughts openly exposed to God Himself and the whole universe too? But this is what will certainly happen when they stand before the final and inescapable throne of judgment. This sobering thought is of the greatest usefulness in bringing forth fruits of worthy repentance. A person should be much more afraid of offending the omnipotent and omniscient Lord of heaven than they should be worried about the fact that other human beings may come to know about their faults and their sins. After all, they themselves know such things to be perfectly true, and also know them to be known to their all-seeing Creator.

And there are those who, strange as it may seem, find themselves disturbed and offended when others say things about them which they themselves are quite willing to accuse themselves of in public.[27] [Paradoxical as it may seem,]

---

[27] The author here seems to be referring to cases where persons will

it is indeed the apex of perfect humility if a person is able to hear others speak of the same faults of which they accuse themselves with undisturbed tranquility, patience, and equanimity! This is a very great and very revealing test of the genuineness of humility. For the one who can do this has attained to real humility, but those who cannot still bear within themselves hidden pride. People who accuse themselves of faults but cannot bear to hear others accusing them of the same faults are, in reality, only seeking to make themselves *seem* righteous and honest—in other words, to make themselves look good! As it is written in Scripture, "[The one who wishes to appear] just is his own first accuser."[28]

---

openly admit some fault or defect within themselves but will then take offence when others point out precisely the same thing about them. This was perhaps a more noticeable occurrence in monasteries where the practice of the "chapter of faults" was observed. During the chapter of faults, monks (or nuns) had the opportunity of confessing their own mistakes or shortcoming to the community and asking for pardon. In many cases, members of the community would then be free to make observations about the faults or errors of their fellow members. Anselm's dwelling on this point at some length in this conference suggests that he may have had certain particular cases in mind when he was speaking.

[28] Proverbs 18:17. Anselm's quotation of the verse here interprets in a slightly unusual, but highly insightful, way. Generally, the verse is taken as signifying that a just person is ready to recognize their own faults. But Anselm interprets it here as indicating that certain people use self-accusation as a means of appearing to be just, or deflecting possible criticism of themselves by others.

For the person who accuses himself but cannot tolerate hearing others accuse him of the same thing—what is he doing except making a show of his own pretensions to humility? But as soon as someone else finds fault with him, he typically accuses those others of falseness or hatred.

If, therefore, anyone wishes to attain to the *real* pinnacle of humility, he should learn to accept others pointing out his faults, especially those faults which he himself is willing to point out about himself. In this way, he will prove himself to possess genuine humility rather than simply having a vain desire to *appear* humble to others.

When such persons arrive at a state of unfeigned and sincere humility, they will look back on their previous life and recognize the wickedness and darkness in which they formerly dwelt. And they will also experience a profound gratitude and ineffable exultation that the light of God's goodness has so kindly illuminated them. They will carefully keep guard of their bodies and they will no less carefully keep guard of their hearts, lest the enemy should seize and steal away the grace which God has bestowed upon them and drag them back into the terrible darkness which they have now left behind. But they will attribute none of the virtues which they have acquired to their own efforts or merits, [but rather to God's grace alone.] Neither shall they consider themselves in any way superior to those who still struggle with sin and have not yet been graced with conversion.

In the advanced level of humility which they have reached, they will govern all their conduct and thoughts with caution. They will hold themselves to be of lesser account and merit than their fellows, not only in words and outward show, but also in the very depths of their heart.[29] "But," you may say, "how is this possible? Take the case of a person who knows (without any pride or exaggeration) that he has the virtues of sobriety, humility, patience, generosity to those in need, and diligence in his service of God, and that he treats others how he would like to be treated himself. Can such a person *really* judge himself to be worse than another who is clearly lustful, proud, dangerous, avaricious, and negligent in their service of God?"

"Yes, indeed!" I confidently reply. For to do otherwise would be to disobey the clear injunctions of Sacred Scripture, which require that we be humble.[30] And no one should presume to imagine that Scripture would ever command us to do anything unless it were actually possible to put it into practice.

Scripture directs the persons who seek after true humility not only to speak of themselves as being less than others but also to believe this sincerely from the very depths of

---

[29] Cf. Rule of St. Benedict 7:51.

[30] Cf. Philippians 2:3.

the heart. Let the mind which is inspired by the Holy Spirit contemplate judiciously how this command may be truly fulfilled!

[But you may object, saying,] "How can a person who is good and holy judge himself, in the innermost depths of his heart, to be truly inferior to a person who has a depraved heart and who does evil works? For both natural and divine law clearly declares that everything and everyone good is, by their very nature, superior to that which is bad or wicked. And, accordingly, virtue and goodness earn a reward of eternal glory, whereas wickedness and vice merit a harvest of unending punishment. But if a person judges anyone who is wicked to be superior to any person who is good (which may well be himself), he is judging falsely and according to a preposterous and perverse mis-ordering of things! And such a judgment would be manifestly contrary both to nature and to simple truth. So the good person who judges himself to be inferior than a wicked person will be flying in the face of truth. But, [on the other hand,] if he does *not* sincerely consider himself to be less than the other, he is disobeying the commandments about humility found in the pages of Sacred Scripture!" [31]

---

[31] Cf. Philippians 2:3, "In humility of mind, let each esteem the other as better than themselves." Anselm also seems to have strongly in mind the *Rule of Benedict* 7:51, that, "one not only declares with his tongue but also believes in his heart that he is inferior to all."

But nothing [of such foolish contentions and paradoxes as these] are to be admitted or accepted! For it is possible both to obey the divine commandment to esteem others as better than oneself without deviating from truth or sincerity. For if any person carefully considers himself, he will be able to determine what is in him which actually comes from himself and what comes to him from the grace of God. And he shall find that there is nothing within himself which originates from himself except for what is bad. Conversely, all the good which he finds within his heart he shall recognize to be a gift from God.[32] Then, in comparing himself to others, he should consider only what is *truly* his own—that is, whatever of wickedness he finds in himself. And he should be mindful always that he may well slip into wickedness himself, whereas the person with whom he is comparing himself may rise to the heights of virtue through the grace of God.

Those who keep such considerations in their heart will never be tempted to extol themselves above others, nor to consider themselves as superior to anyone else. On the contrary, the more closely and lovingly a person adheres to God in his heart, the more humble he will become in

[32] Cf. *Rule of Benedict* 4:41–42. "If you notice something good in yourself, attribute it to the grace of God and not to yourself. But be sure that whatever wickedness you commit is always of your own doing, and should be attributed to yourself alone."

evaluating his own merits, and the less prone he will be to condemning others. For he shall recognize that all his brothers and sisters in the human family are also beloved children of God, created by Him and dear to Him. Thus through true love of God, true humility is attained, and through true humility, true love of one's neighbor.

Eadmer's Concluding Note to Brother William

THE WORDS WHICH you have read above are those which I received from the mouth of our holy father, Anselm, and which I have diligently written down. This I have done out of a desire to satisfy you, my friend, who have requested that I should commit these words of Anselm to paper.

The letter at the beginning has been added so that anyone who might read this work will not have cause to wonder at the discrepancy between the beauty of the ideas [which are Anselm's] and the unpolished and unlearned nature of the writing and expression [which is my own.] For otherwise, the reader should certainly conclude that Anselm himself is the author when they consider the refinement and elegance of the ideas. But, [if they assumed that this was the case,] they would certainly marvel that such a learned man has somehow apparently lost his accustomed clarity and eloquence!

However, whoever reads this small work should be assured that Anselm himself has often read this draft which I have prepared, and also heard it read aloud to him. And he has given his full approval and authorization of the work and directed that it should be copied and circulated freely so that future generations may read it.

May God be blessed in all things! Amen.

MEDITATION ON THE DAY OF JUDGMENT AND THE BLESSINGS OF HEAVEN

WHAT, I ASK you, is there in this present existence which could possibly compare to the blessings and gifts which God shall offer us in the future? A little reflection will show that there is nothing amongst the good things of this present life which remotely approaches the magnitude and splendor of the joys which the blessed souls possess in heaven.

The beginning of our future life coincides with the end of our present life—and both of these coincide with the moment of physical death. Does not nature itself seem to abhor death? Is there any living creature which does not fear it in some way or another? For if we look at any of the animals, they will take to flight or conceal themselves in some hiding place whenever some danger which puts their life in peril approaches them. They will try to avoid death in such ways and a thousand others!

But you, O my soul, if you find this earthly life to be a time of labor and trial, if you know the burdens and anxieties of earthly cares, or if you have experienced the many pains and discomforts of this mortal flesh—should you not rather regard death as a blessing, or at least not a thing to be dreaded? For the moment of death brings with it a cessation of all earthly cares. It relieves the heart of all burdens and puts to rest all the discomfort and pains of the mortal body. In this respect, is it not more desirable than all earthly honors and riches, and more pleasing than all pleasures and joys?

If you have a serene and untroubled conscience and if you have certain hope of the future life, you will not fear death in the least. This is the experience most of all for those who, whilst straining under the servitude of this mortal life, find their minds often raised up in contemplation to the glories of heaven. These times of celestial contemplation are the sweet preludes of the future beatitude of paradise. Through such preludes and foretastes of the bliss of our celestial homeland, faith is able to overcome one's natural and instinctive fear of death. Hope conquers this fear, and a clean conscience puts it to flight.

For a soul who is armed with such faith, hope, and serenity of conscience, death appears as the beginning of a longed-for rest and the happy termination of the time of labor. Thus it is written, "Blessed are the dead, who have died in the Lord."[1] But the prophet Isaiah makes a very clear distinction between the death of the wicked (which is a source of horror to them) and the death of the just (which is a source of peace and consolation). He declares, "All kings shall go to their merited resting place and each soul shall go to dwell in its fitting home. But you wicked shall be cast from your tombs like unfruitful branches, polluted and twisted!"[2]

Those whose death is commended by a good conscience will go to rest in glory, for "precious in the eyes of the Lord is the death of his faithful."[3] They shall indeed sleep in blessedness. Hosts of angels will be present at their passing from this life. The saints will rush to greet them. All of these, the angels and saints, shall become their fellow citizens in the heavenly city. These angels and saints shall comfort and defend the soul of the just and faithful person in his hour of death. They shall fight against the multitude of demons who attempt to seize upon each soul as it passes from the tenement of its mortal body. They shall refute the wicked spirits who accuse it, and will thus lead it to

---

1 Revelation 14:13.

2 Isaiah 14:18–19.

3 Psalm 115:15.

the bosom of holy Abraham and guide it into the celestial kingdom of everlasting peace.

But, alas, it shall not be thus for the wicked! Rather, at the time of mortal death, their souls shall go forth from their bodies like a foul stench issuing from an open grave. Diabolical spirits will hasten to seize it with their infernal instruments of torture, and the soul itself will be found to be polluted and befouled with hidden lusts and wicked desires. In its realm of torment, hellish birds shall tear at it, and the fetid gales and oppressive miasmas of the underworld shall suffocate it.

Truly, "the inheritance of the just is joy, but the hopes of the wicked shall perish."[4] No words are able to express the nature and quality of that eternal rest, of that perfect peace, of the infinite joy in the bosom of Abraham, which is promised to those who depart from this world in true faith. It exceeds anything we have ever experienced, and anything we can imagine. All the souls of the blessed shall be united with their loved ones in paradise, joyfully awaiting the Day of Final Judgment, when they are to be united once more with their bodies and clothed with the radiant garments of immortality and glory.

***

[4] Proverbs 10;28

But consider now, my soul, the awesome terror of that impending Day of Judgment. The firmament of the skies shall tremble, and the vault of heaven shake. The elements of the earth shall be dissolved in fire, and the underworld shall be torn open. All things that are now hidden and secret—words, thoughts, and deeds—will then be clearly revealed. And the Lord shall appear as a judge, borne upon the chariot of a tempest[5] and armed with His burning fury. In His divine anger, He will deal out retribution and bring forth devastation as a consuming fire. Blessed are those who are ready for that day and have taken due care that their souls are well prepared! But what will happen then to those wretched souls who have been negligent and careless and allowed themselves to be enmeshed in sin? What then of those who now wallow in lust, who waste themselves in avarice and exult themselves in arrogant pride? Most assuredly, they shall be miserable on that day! "The angels will go forth, and separate the wicked from the good,"[6] the latter standing at the right hand of God's glorious throne of splendor and the former assembling at the left.[7]

My soul, imagine yourself to be present at that tremendous Day of Judgment! Consider yourself not yet judged, and not yet directed either to stand rejoicing amongst the

---

[5] Cf. Jeremiah 4:13.

[6] Matthew 13:49.

[7] Cf. Matthew 25:33.

sheep at the right of God's throne nor sent to suffer at the left with the goats. Look firstly to the crowd who are at the left side of the eternal Judge. Behold their dire and abject misery! How much horror, how much shame, how much foulness, how much pain is there! They stand trembling, wretched and forlorn, grinding their teeth, striking their chests, horrible in visage, contorted in pain, utterly confused and confounded. They desire to hide, but there is nowhere to hide. They long to flee, but they stand immobile and fixed. If they turn their eyes upwards, they behold the terrifying countenance and awesome majesty of their divine Judge. If they turn their eyes downwards, they see the abyss, the bottomless pit of the inferno! No excuses for crimes and sins will then be permitted or accepted. Neither will the judgment of God be in any way able to be swayed by clever arguments or persuasions. For each person's conscience shall be opened up, and plainly visible to all. Not only the actions but the intentions and motivations of each and every person will stand clearly exposed and be indisputably and manifestly evident.

Now, my soul, turn your eyes to the right, and behold there the glories which shall be yours if you find yourself numbered amongst this assembly of the blessed! How much beauty is there, how much honor, how much happiness, how much security! Some of those who are amongst this number of the blessed shall be seated upon splendid thrones of power. Others will be glorified with the radiant crown of martyrdom. Yet others will be splendid and graceful with the angelic beauty of unstained virginity. There will be those who are adorned with the generosity of almsgiving, and those who bear the noble decorations of learning and wisdom. And this entire assembly, though diverse in its multitude of splendors and virtues, shall be harmoniously united in a perfect bond of ineffable charity. The face of Jesus will shine upon them, not as the terrifying countenance of a strict judge, but as a loveable and loving shepherd; not as bitterness, but as sweetness; not as something to be dreaded, but as something to be adored.

Imagine yourself to be standing thus before the Throne of Judgment and to have examined the crowds on its two sides—those on the left, the damned, in their misery and pain, and those on the right, the blessed, in their happiness and glory. As for yourself, imagine that the side to which *you* are to go has not yet been announced. How anxiously you await to hear the eternal sentence which you have merited! You may well say to yourself then, "Trembling comes over me, and darkness overshadows me."[8]

Act now, act now, my soul, to ensure that it goes well for you on that final day.

***

---

[8] Psalm 54:6.

O Lord, if You send me to the left to be numbered amongst the damned, I know that I will have no grounds for disputing with Your judgment, for I confess that I am a sinner. And if You send me to the right, it shall be thanks to Your mercy and love alone, not due to any merits of my own. Thus truly, O Lord, my life and my eternal destiny lies in Your will!

Therefore, each one who finds themselves to be counted among the blessed on the final day ought to be filled with a tremendous love of God and gratitude towards Him. Imagine your joy when you hear it said to you, "Come to Me, ye blessed of My Father, receive the kingdom which has been prepared for you since the beginning of time!" But that dreaded sentence will resonate like grim thunder in the ears of the damned, "Depart from Me, ye accursed, into the fire which is never extinguished." And then the wicked shall go off to everlasting punishment, while the just shall enter into eternal life.[9] Irrevocable then will be the sentence, and inexorable will be the judgment!

The worst of all the multitude of the punishments and torments which shall afflict the condemned is the knowledge that they have been deprived forever and definitively from the glory of the vision of God. But as for the blessed, they will be enrolled amongst the glorious orders of the angels and saints in accordance with their grade and

---

9 Cf. Matthew 25:34–46.

merits. And what a wonderful and magnificent procession that shall be, with Christ Himself as the head and leader, followed by all others in their proper order. And they shall enter the kingdom of God the Father, there to reign with Him eternally, receiving the kingdom which has been prepared for them since the beginning of the world. No one is able to comprehend or imagine the immensity and glory of this kingdom, much less to express it in words! In this kingdom, there shall be nothing lacking, of all that the hearts of humans or angels, or even of God Himself, could possibly desire!

There will be naught there of mourning, no weeping, no tears, no pain, no fear. Neither will there be any sadness, nor discord, nor envy, nor ambition. Trial and tribulation, trouble and temptation will be gone forever. Death and old age, sickness and poverty will all be consigned to oblivion, forgotten, and never to return.

O my soul, when all these afflictions are removed—when there shall be no trace of sorrow or sadness, of trial or tribulation, of suffering or sin—what will remain but pure and unalloyed joy? Where there is no longer any strife or strain or struggle or stress, what will there be but total tranquility and perfect peace? When there is no longer anything to fear, what shall there be but utter security and unassailable safety? When there is no longer the need to toil nor any possible affliction or deficiency, what will there be but invincible strength and immortal well-being? Where all darkness and shadow has been utterly and finally banished and expelled, what will there be but pure and perfect light, the ineffable and inconceivable radiance of heaven's glory? And when death and mortality has been vanquished forever, what shall there be but eternal life?

What more could we desire or seek than all of these blessings, than this plenitude of perfect beatitude? We have attempted to describe it, but truly it is utterly beyond all powers of description.

Yet there is one thing which shall exceed even these blessings and boons—and that is the vision of God, the knowledge of God and the love of God. It is only then that God shall be seen, known, and loved as He really is. The souls of the blessed shall behold God in His purity and in His essence, in His magnitude and in His magnificence. How loving shall be His face, and how adorable and desirable His countenance! It is this glorious face of God that the legions of seraphim and the host of angels desire so ardently to gaze upon. Who can describe its plenitude, its light, it sweetness?

The Father shall be seen in the Son, and the Son will be made visible in the Father. The Holy Spirit, the living flame of love, shall be manifest in both. The glorious Trinity will at last be perceived in its fullness and absolute reality. It was of this beautiful vision of the Triune Deity that Our

Lord spoke when He said, "The one who loves me shall be loved by my Father, and I will love him, and make myself manifest to him."[10]

Out of this wondrous vision of the Trinity, perfect knowledge of God will arise. Of this mystical and deifying knowledge, it is written, "This is eternal life: that they shall know that you alone are God."[11] And out of this glorious vision and knowledge of God, the greatest thing of all will arise—the perfect love for God. This shall be an eternal fire of divine love, the ineffable sweetness of sanctified and sanctifying charity. No desire shall be unfulfilled, yet no satiety shall inhibit or make dull the flame of holy desire.

What, you may ask, is this stupendous and glorious mystery which we have attempted to describe? My soul, it is indeed that which "eye has not seen, nor ear heard, nor the human mind conceived—that which God has prepared for all those who love him!"[12]

---

[10] John 14:21.
[11] John 17:3.
[12] 1 Corinthians 2:9.

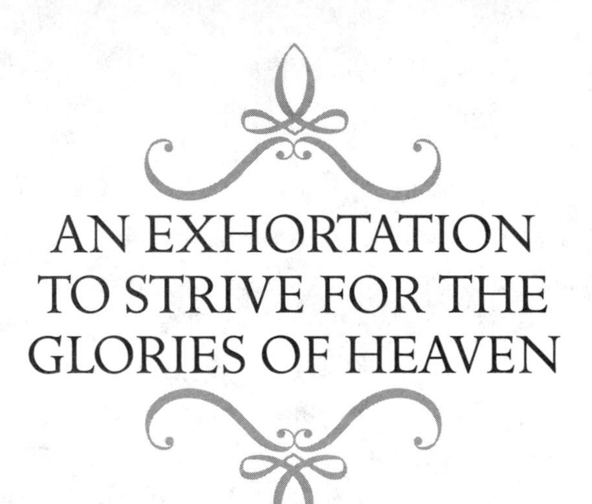

AN EXHORTATION TO STRIVE FOR THE GLORIES OF HEAVEN

My friend, what is it that you are doing? Why is it that, like a beast, you immerse yourself so enthusiastically and avidly in the vain and ephemeral things of this passing world? The Lord has created you as a rational and intelligent being. Do not make yourself like those brute animals who lack this wonderful faculty and who are bereft of the reason and wisdom with which you are blessed! Wake up! O pitiful one, have pity on yourself! Act like the rational being which God created you to be. It was on your account that God, the Most High, descended from His heavenly kingdom to be incarnate upon this earth as our divine Savior. And He did this for no other reason than that He might raise you up to heaven to be with Him and to share His eternal glory and beatitude.

My friend, you have been invited as a special guest to the wedding banquet of your celestial Spouse. Why do you stubbornly neglect this marvelous invitation and show yourself unworthy of it? And how do you expect to enter into this glorious, eternal wedding feast when you have not bothered to prepare a suitable garment for yourself, nor lighted your lamp in readiness? Remember that this present world is but a fleeting and deceptive dream and shadow which shall soon pass. Direct your thoughts and your longings instead to that which is eternal—to God and to heaven. Cleanse yourself from all malice, worldly desire, and sin, and let your affections yearn instead for the pure love of your divine Redeemer.

Restrain yourself in all earthly things. Emulate the angels, and strive to make all your thoughts and desires chaste and holy. Correct any sinful thoughts as soon as they arise, and do not let yourself become engrossed in earthly schemes and endeavors. Free your soul from the chains which bind it to the passing vanities of this material realm—avarice, lust, and ambition. For when you attain to liberty from all that ties you to the earth, you shall truly be crowned by Christ and given a glorious place above the very firmament of heaven. In the meantime, you should imitate the clouds which float above the skies, giving forth abundant rain in the form of sincere tears of compunction. When this saving rain falls—that is, the tears of true penitence—it shall unfailingly serve to extinguish all the pernicious flames of sin which lurk and smolder within your heart.

***

It is wise frequently to call to mind the dreadful Day of Judgment. For, though we do not know when it shall come, we *do* know that it is approaching inexorably and unavoidably. Seek now to find suitable remedies for all the wounds of sin which you bear. Walk strongly and with firm constancy in the law of the Lord. Make yourself into a worthy temple of the Holy Spirit by faith and charity. Strive to grow a little in virtue every day, always inspired by the sure hope of seeing the Lord God in the radiant splendor and indescribable joy of His eternal kingdom.

But take care to shun idle gossip and empty conversation lest you unwittingly stray from the commands of Christ. Plant in your heart and soul the seeds of goodness. These seeds of goodness are the virtues, as wonderfully exemplified by the holy fathers and saints and all those who have served God faithfully through the ages.

And remember that, in this present life, the path which you must walk is strewn with the snares and traps of the devil! Be vigilant lest you fall into one of his many lethal pits. Always bear in mind that your life on earth will not be very long, even if you live to the very maximum number of years possible for a mortal. You cannot be certain when death will arrive; do not assume that you will have time to repent at some point in the future, for you do not know when your end will come. Remain always fixed on Christ so that your yearnings and desires may be holy and pure. In this way, your soul will become like a fruitful vine, and your life shall be rendered pleasing and acceptable to the God Who created you.

Always keep before the eyes of your mind your final day, when death shall arrive like a thief in the night. Strive to be ready and prepared to depart from this world at all times so that you may be found clean from sin and free of guilt on that fateful day. In this way, you may ensure that your soul shall ascend to God and to the bliss of heaven, borne by the hands of the holy angels and accompanied by the noble company of saints.

***

My friend, it is well for you to regard all the things of this earth with a measure of detachment and even disdain. Do not cling to them, but direct your desire and your love to your Redeemer. Be ever mindful of your soul and its eternal destiny. For those things which seem most sweet and delightful in this life often serve as the snares of the devil. And if you permit yourself to become enmeshed in his insidious snares, on your final day you will find yourself confronted with an overwhelming anxiety. Truly, if you find yourself in a state of sin on the day of your death, your soul shall then wither and be left trembling with very fear!

Always be ready, my friend! Never cease to remind yourself of the vanity and insufficiency of all earthly things. None of these can bring the soul true satisfaction or enduring happiness. Restrain yourself from all unbecoming and shameful thoughts. Arouse yourself from the sleep of sin and the dullness of iniquity! If you truly desire the glories of heaven and the happiness which is eternal, treat with disdain all passing pleasures and all time-bound glories. Follow the noble example of the saints, who have themselves already merited eternal beatitude. By emulating the paths they walked, you shall also arrive at the celestial homeland of everlasting delight.

O miserable wretch, why do you so often behave as if you cared nothing for your true life and your eternal destiny? Why do you so foolishly neglect the fate of your immortal soul? Hurry! Take action now while you still have the opportunity to repent, before the door to unending bliss is closed to you. Your repentance will not only obtain eternal life for you but shall bring delight and rejoicing to the whole heavenly host of saints and angels.

Your divine Physician, Christ, is patiently waiting for your tears of repentance. Draw near to Him; do not fear! Reveal to Him, your heavenly Doctor, each of the secret wounds of sin and vice which you bear. For these can all readily be healed with the balm of tears and the ointment of compunction. The door of repentance is still wide open to you, my friend. Hasten to it! Run, and run quickly; run with all your strength and all your determination—before it is closed to you forever.

While there is yet time, pour out tears of sincere repentance. For it is infinitely better that you should mourn in this present world than that you should mourn eternally in the world to come. Now, there is mercy; in that next world, there shall be only exacting judgment. Here, one may often find some pleasures in sin, but in the next world, only their torments shall remain. Here, one may easily laugh, but in the world to come, many will weep, and weep inconsolably and perpetually. Here, many enjoy the sounds of music, but in hell, there will be nothing but eternal fire. Here, many clad themselves in fine vestments and rich garments; in hell, there shall be nothing but the gnawing of that dreaded worm which never dies and the searing heat of that horrendous flame which is never extinguished!

Therefore, my friend, repent in this present life while you still have the opportunity so that you may avoid being condemned to the outer darkness. Let no earthly and fleshly pleasures delight you or enthrall you; rather, strive to see them as the bitter and empty deceptions which they are.

Alas, we are all sinners, and all tepid in our faith. Who is there who would not weep for us and feel pity for our ignorance and feebleness? It is as if we care nothing for eternal life, but love death with all our hearts!

What could be more noble and more magnificent than to raise our minds and desires up to the heights of heaven? To do this, we must first train and discipline our body so that it accepts its proper role of a servant and becomes obedient to the commands of the soul. Only thus will it be ready and willing to put into practice the good intentions of our minds. What more delightful and satisfying dish is there than to do the will of God? And what is more exhilarating than to overcome the power of the devil through strength of mind?

Whoever truly conquers their own self will be able to restrain the impulses of wrath, sloth, lust, and greed. Such persons shall not be led astray by any fleshly temptations or earthly blandishments. They shall not be perturbed by adversity, nor will they be inflated when things go well for them. They shall not be blown around by the winds of change which never cease to blow in this inconstant and capricious world. Consider in your own self what is better—to repent for your sins in this present life and perhaps to forgo some of the insubstantial and passing pleasures of vice or to weep forever, and to lament in vain, in the eternal fires of hell?

***

Why do you let the powers and energies of your soul be dissipated and wasted by pursuing so avidly the perishable things of this passing world? Instead, elevate your mind to the glorious radiance of everlasting happiness, to those wondrous and magnificent things which eye has not seen, nor ear heard, which God has prepared for all those who love him.[1] Learn to control your tongue. Exercise diligent restraint over your eyes, your eating, your dress, your thoughts, and your laughter. In this way, you shall exhibit yourself to all as a perfect athlete of God! Do your best to make no enemies for yourself. Rather, strive to have only one foe—that is, the devil.

What does it benefit you to gain some high or exalted position if it brings you more concerns and anxieties? What real happiness do you gain from fine vestments or garments? If you are promoted to a position of dignity or responsibility, why be inflated with pride? It behooves such a person more to tremble with fear, knowing that their actions and omissions will be seen more clearly and judged more exactingly, both by humans and by angels. Why do you persist in sinning, and therefore sadden your heavenly Father, Who has graciously deigned to count you amongst His beloved children?

Hold back your tongue from all evil. Seek peace and pursue it.[2] Do not make your divine Lord and Master angry with you, lest He regard you as a wicked servant deserving of punishment. Instead, follow Him to the glory to which

1 Cf. 1 Corinthians 2:9.

2 Cf. Psalm 33:14

He has so lovingly invited you! Prepare yourself to obey the orders of your eternal King, even if it means denying your own self-will at times. Be content with all that is simple, poor, and lowly, and be happy to find yourself in the last place. Be humble not only in speech but in your very thoughts. Commit yourself to doing in the here and now whatever will profit you for all eternity.

Arise in the hours of the night to pour forth private prayers and tears to God. Implore Him to liberate you from the snares and stumbling blocks of the carnal passions. Imagine that your soul was to be suddenly seized away from you. How would it be judged at this very moment? Would it be found to be polluted with sin and negligent of its duty of repentance? If you were to speak to your own self at your moment of death, what advice would you give? Always have this moment of death before your eyes. In what state do you wish to be found when you face the dreaded and inexorable Day of Judgment? My friend, do *now* whatever is necessary to achieve such a state. Fill your lamp now with the oil of the virtues and ensure that it is lighted and ready with the fire of charity and faith.

Treat with detachment all things which are temporal and passing. Disregard the pomps and pretensions of this world. Like a warrior preparing for a fierce battle, focus on nothing but obtaining the great reward of victory! Flee to your own conscience for advice. And unburden yourself from your earthly cares and solicitudes. Do not let contention, stubbornness, or self-will reign within your heart, and never let vice dominate you. Disdain what is earthly and desire what is heavenly; renounce the joys which are passing and cling instead to that happiness which endures forever.

Rouse yourself from your woeful sleepiness and torpor. Open your mouth and pray to God that He may, in His great mercy, free you from the burden of your sins. Pray frequently, and do not cease to let tears of repentance flow, either from your eyes or in your heart. Shun feebleness of soul, deplore whatever negligence you find in yourself, and abhor all your sins and vices. But cultivate mercy, and learn to love self-restraint. Pray the holy psalms diligently, and let them lead you to the peaceful fields of holy meditation.

Make haste to pray while you yet have time, and do not delay repenting for your sins. Be reconciled to God while you still have the chance of doing so easily! Love God with all your heart, for that is how God loves you. Fear the Day of Judgment, and keep careful guard over all the actions of your life. Strive to make yourself a stranger to the affairs of this passing world so that you may cling more diligently to the kingdom of God.

***

Listen carefully, my soul, and give ear to what I say to you. Attend diligently to my warnings. Do not permit yourself to become polluted with anything unclean, and do not let yourself be stained by the foulness of vice and lust. Strive to hold yourself above all fleshly corruption, and resist all the impulses and drives which are purely bestial within yourself. Let neither lust nor the desire for pleasure conquer you or rule you. Indeed, it is better to die than to become polluted with lust! It is better to let the soul go forth from the body entirely than to be reduced to being a prisoner and slave of the impulses of the flesh.

Chastity makes a human being close to God, and it also makes God come close to that human being. For the kingdom of God is promised to those of chaste and pure hearts. If you ever find that you are affected by the stings and temptations of lust and distracted and disturbed by the urgings of the flesh, think at once of the day of your death. Place the grim hour of your passing from this mortal life before the eyes of your mind. Call to mind the future judgment and the unspeakable torments which await the souls who are damned. Imagine the perpetual fires of hell and the horrible pains of Gehenna. Such thoughts will certainly subdue the promptings of lust most effectively!

Pray ceaselessly, with tears of compunction and earnestness. Apply yourself to prayer insistently and frequently. Implore the Lord for mercy and protection day and night. And even when you close your eyes to sleep, continue to pray.

For frequent prayer disarms all the spears and weapons of the devil. It drives out unclean spirits and conquers demons. Indeed, prayer prevails against evils of every kind.

Never fully appease the appetites of the body, lest they come to dominate you. Do not eat to satiety, but only to sufficiency. Discipline your body by being sparing with it, cultivating the helpful practices of fasting and abstinence. Be prepared to feel a little hunger and thirst, for such things are healthy and salubrious, both to soul and body. Learn to abstain and to say no to the appetites and impulses of your flesh! Unless you have learnt to fast at times, you will have little chance of resisting any more substantial and subtle temptations.

Be humble, and let yourself be founded in humility. In all your action, follow the example of those who are righteous, and even try to imitate the saints and angels. Let nothing in this passing world shock or upset you, nor be the source of sadness or despondency to you. Seek not for popular acclaim or public glory. Try to *be* good rather than to *be seen* as being good.

My friend, why do you put off enacting your good resolutions until tomorrow? You are able to gain for yourself that which you desire—that is, virtue and its rewards—this very day! But remember that virtue and innocence, though gained only through long and patient discipline, can all be lost within a single hour.

***

The pleasures, joys, and honors of this mortal life are but brief and ephemeral. They fly away from us like the wind; they vanish like shadows; they are blown away like smoke. Earthly power is always fragile and uncertain. Consider all the great people of the past—the kings, the princes, the potentates, the rich, the learned. Where are they all now? In the same place—the grave! They have passed away like fleeting shadows; they have vanished like insubstantial dreams.

Earthly cares and responsibilities burden and vex the mind. If you wish to experience tranquility and peace, do not aspire for the things of this world. But your mind will always be at peace if you can cast off earthly cares and desires. Whatever enmeshes you in the things of this world and binds you to the visible and temporal realm separates you, to some degree or another, from the love of God and from the things which are eternal.

For no one can aspire to the glory of God and at the same time cling to the glory of this passing world. No one can embrace both Christ and the world at the same time. Since God is all and everything, be ready to renounce all and everything for the sake God. Strive to serve God unfettered by any mortal bonds.

Give everything to God, and present all that you are to His service. For what God shall give you will be much greater than what you give Him! The gratitude God will exhibit to you will far exceed any gift you offer Him.

My friend, endeavor to become a temple of God so that the Spirit of the Most High may dwell within you. Serve the poor and needy according to the fullest extent of your capacities. Do not take from anyone anything which you do not intend to bestow upon another.

Whatever you do in this present life, do it with your future and everlasting reward in mind. Look forward with holy desire to the wages of eternal life and everlasting beatitude. For it is a future reward that is promised to the saints, not any recompense in this present life. The reward of righteousness and sanctity is not to be found on earth but in heaven. We should not seek to find perfect happiness and peace here in this earthly valley of tears, for it is promised to us only in another realm, in the star-girt kingdom of the celestial Jerusalem!

Act and think now as if you are dead to the world, and let the world be dead to you. Look at the glories of this passing sphere as if you were already amongst the dead and had left all mortal cares and aspirations far behind. Imagine that you are already resting in your tomb, and that the wealth, honor, and pleasure of this terrestrial orb mean nothing to you. Do not allow your heart to be infatuated with anything from which you are destined to be separated, either sooner or later. For whatever you are not able to possess eternally, you never truly possess at all.

Do nothing for the sake of obtaining merely human praise, or popular acclaim, or public fame. For such things involve much effort and anxiety, but they are really nothing at all. Instead, do everything for the sake of the eternal life and the everlasting and unbounded happiness of heaven, which—if you but act justly, love tenderly, and believe sincerely—Christ, in His infinite mercy and love, shall most assuredly bestow upon you; Who, with the Father and the Holy Spirit, lives and reigns forever and ever. Amen.